Trends in Mental Health
Evaluation

Trends in Mental Health Evaluation

Elizabeth Warren Markson
Massachusetts Department of
Mental Health

David Franklyn Allen
Massachusetts Department of
Mental Health

Lexington Books
D.C. Heath and Company
Lexington, Massachusetts
Toronto   London

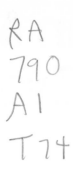

RA
790
A1
T74

Library of Congress Cataloging in Publication Data

Main entry under title:
 Trends in mental health evaluation.

 "This book is an outgrowth of the first New England Conference on
Evaluation of Mental Health Services, held in Boston in May 1975."
 1. Mental health services—Evaluations—Congresses. I. Markson, Eliza-
beth Warren. II. Allen, David Franklyn.
RA790.A1T74   362.2   75-32869
ISBN 0-699-00367-0

International Standard Book Number: 0-669-00367-0

Library of Congress Catalog Card Number: 75-32869

To
Clifford Beers
and
Dorothea Dix

Contents

List of Figures

List of Tables

Foreword

As the mental health "data pile" continues to grow, the evaluation literature begins to parallel it: diffuse, random, unintegrated, and unsynthesized. This book hopefully represents a beginning attempt to remedy the situation. An earlier effort to focus attention on this state of affairs led to a conference in 1970 held in Philadelphia on "Evaluation of Community Mental Health Centers" (CMHC). It was the first scientific conference of the fledgling National Council of Community Mental Health Centers. Sponsored by the National Institute of Mental Health (NIMH), it convened the first national gathering of CMHC leadership. Both macroscopic and microscopic expositions of different approaches to similar evaluation problems were illustrated by methodologies being developed in four large urban centers.

Over the past few years these information and evaluation systems have been debugged and are functioning relatively well. Trial and error have modified them. They are illustrative of similar experiences with mental health program evaluation at the national, state, and local levels. The time has now come to evaluate the effects of these efforts between and across systems.

It is interesting to reflect on some of the observations and recommendations that emerged from the Philadelphia conference over five years ago. A theme that received a great deal of attention was "the atmosphere for evaluation." Elaborations of this theme were: attitudes of commitment to disinterested, open, empirical study and review of ongoing programs; mechanisms for the facilitation and stimulation of priority for assessment and program validation by both clinicians and administrators; traditions of involvement or resistance to evaluation by professionals.

Another recurrent topic was that evaluation cannot meaningfully exist outside the overt and covert matrix of objectives and goals. This issue emphasized the symbiosis between ongoing rational planning processes and integrated program evaluation research.

The paucity of training for evaluation was a point frequently made. The need to develop an expert cadre of behavioral scientists able to operate as evaluators both intramurally and extramurally was stressed. The critical nature of evaluation research demands maximum participation by all concerned parties in both planning and execution of evaluative strategies and therefore requires that the evaluators be trained in the skills necessary to facilitate this. Emphasis on the ability to be part of and yet outside the program or system being studied underscored the personality requirements for evaluators in terms of tolerance for resistance and ambiguity and skills in tension reduction.

In keeping with the need for pluralism in approaching evaluation from both the methodological as well as the stylistic point of view, concern was voiced as to the discrepancies in evaluation potential among rural and urban systems.

Discussion also ranged over the hazards of "creeping" erosion of privacy and confidentiality; questions of stabilizing support by earmarking funds for evaluation; development of increasingly sophisticated tools for program assessment. Creating a multidisciplinary resource pool of expert consultants reaching beyond mental health into economics, law, urban planning, etc.

In reading the points raised by the persons interested in community mental health evaluation in 1970, we must ask whether this quasi evaluation, or assessment of the state of the art, had any impact. The answer may well be one of cautious optimism on at least one manifest level of public response. In the Community Mental Health Centers Amendments of 1975 (Title III of PL 94-63) Congress mandates a percentage of funds to be allocated for program evaluation. The legislation creates a two-tiered system with not less than 2 percent of a center's operating costs "for a program of continuing evaluation of the effectiveness of its programs in serving the needs of the residents of its catchment area and for a review of the quality of the services provided by the center. . . ." HEW may utilize up to 1 percent of the appropriation for grants under the Act for contracts or grants for evaluation. John Cumming, in Chapter 7, analyzes the multiple implications of this development.

The contributions of Carol Weiss and Gary Tischler address themselves to the central theme of how evaluators position themselves, utilize their tools, and maximize their leverage in the system they are studying.

The refining of evaluation methodology, though still relatively embryonic, is addressed by Marcia Guttentag, Theodore Kiresuk (a participant in the 1970 conference), and Jean Endicott and Robert Spitzer. Representing some of the more advanced evaluation researchers in the field, they provide encouragement as to the potential for refinement of increasingly sophisticated instruments.

Herbert Schulberg, Lee Macht, Edgar Casper, Elaine Cumming, and Elizabeth Markson raise questions, pose issues, and reflect on problems and unfinished business. Dave Allen, out of his unique experience with field assessment and program evaluation of total catchment area service networks, adds the dimension of ethical considerations in evaluation. Such concerns reflect, at least, a sign of the growing maturation of evaluative research.

All, however, is not progress. What of the issues raised about training and appropriate work force development? There remains a conspicuous absence of allocation of training resources to the development of professional evaluative researchers. Equally important, there has been little or no effort to integrate understanding, receptiveness, and sensitivity to evaluation into mental health graduate and professional training or to formalize any continuing education in evaluation for the field at large. Though often recommended to the NIMH, this agency has failed to give significant priority to this area and has still not initiated the development of an intramural evaluation research laboratory on a par with clinical and biomedical in-house laboratories.

Similarly, as the gap between new knowledge and its utilization continues to widen, only slight attention has been given to information dissemination. This is not to minimize the excellent efforts initiated by Howard Davis in effecting the publication of two journals by NIMH, *Evaluation* and *Innovations*. Likewise, Saul Feldman's inauguration of the journal *Administration in Mental Health* is relevant. True, much of the work reported in this book has been supported by NIMH; yet the very fact that this publication, the first of its kind, has waited until 1976 to be published underscores the relative neglect the field has suffered. It is not by chance that Congress stipulated precise commitments to community mental health program evaluation.

Certainly it is tempting at first blush to react cynically to an evaluation of current effects of previous or ongoing mental health evaluation. All too numerous instances of the seeming imperviousness of an ossified mental health system spring to mind. For instance, why have day and night treatment and rehabilitation services remained underdeveloped as a valid and in some cases preferable alternative to hospitalization, in spite of the growing mass of data attesting to the validity of such options and their economies? It will be interesting to note the impact on health practices in general of the new information on the effects of basic habits of living, e.g., hours of sleep, eating patterns, exercise, weight, drinking, etc., which influence morbidity and longevity far more than any corrective, pathology-reparative efforts. My guess is that once again the lay public and legislators will show greater responsiveness to these data than will the health establishment.

Increased demands for evaluative information will be made as economic constraints force unpleasant and previously avoided choices on government decisionmakers and as the rate of expansion of human services resources constricts. It is in the nature of our work that results appear slowly. This will not, however, diminish the insistence for differentiating information from authorities both within and without government. It is therefore incumbent upon us both to resist premature conclusions and simultaneously to enhance our capability for "action" research. This must be concise, narrowly focused, brief in duration, well defined, and of necessity impressionistic.

We must be careful to discriminate between the varied motivations that maintain pressure for evaluative data. It seems fair to expect that the full spectrum of reasons will accompany such requests. Hopefully we will see a concomitant growth of rational, objective input into program planning and managerial decisionmaking. What we have to guard against most is the denial of complexity in human service programs, in general, and the resultant negativism and tyranny of simplistic solutions.

William Goldman

Preface

This book is an outgrowth of the first New England Conference on Evaluation of Mental Health Services, held in Boston in May 1975. The conference was organized by the Massachusetts Department of Mental Health and supported in part by a contract from NIMH. The conference brought together nationally known experts in the field with local evaluators in the New England states to exchange ideas and discuss general problems in evaluation as well as ones specific to various programs in the agencies represented.

The major reason for this conference, as well as for this book, is its subject population—those people receiving some form of mental health services. The proliferation of services, the recent emphasis on community-based treatment, the reaffirmation of right to treatment (as in *Wyatt v. Stickney*), and congressional mandates for evaluation of treatment have all combined to create a situation where evaluation in mental health is no longer a luxury but a necessity.

Yet the field of evaluation is still relatively young. This itself presents a challenge to be met not only for dissemination of existing knowledge but also by assessment of some of the very real needs and problems surrounding the process of evaluative research.

Not intended as an all-inclusive handbook of evaluation, this book attempts rather to give an overview of a few current policies, techniques, and problems in mental health evaluation. The emergent nature of evaluation would seem to demand the kind of eclectic approach obvious in this collection of papers. Because of the lack of consensus about mental health and evaluation, there is no large scientific body of knowledge that may be drawn upon to provide systematic directives for measurement of successful delivery of mental health service.

The editors of this book have been prompted by an action-research orientation. We began with the premise that good programs in mental health are desirable and much needed. We also assumed that evaluation is a tool which may assist development and assurance of appropriate quality care to everyone who needs it. Past experience in human services has indicated that good intentions in treatment are not enough. The usefulness of mental health services eventually must be measured not in terms of the good intentions or qualifications of those delivering care but rather in terms of outcome—whether what was done produced the desired result in the target population. Furthermore, it is a poorly affordable gamble to assess mental health services only in terms of the time and dollars expended; the "benefit" side of the now famous cost-benefit ratio must be emphasized heavily.

We hope this collection of articles will be of interest to those concerned with program evaluation, whether from a research, monitoring, or policy view.

We should like to thank Richard Elwell, Leon Nicks, and Brian Flynn, Region

I, NIMH, for their encouragement and support in the planning for the conference from which this book stemmed. Dale Levine contributed a fine editorial hand that did much to polish the manuscript and also typed it. Finally, we are grateful to the contributors for making this book a reality and its preparation a rewarding experience.

Elizabeth W. Markson
David Allen

Part I:
Bases and Policies for
Evaluation

1

Mental Health Programs, Past, Present, and Future: Bases for Evaluation

Lee B. Macht

The purpose of this first chapter is to provide some of the program bases for the following chapters on evaluation per se. It will outline some of the history of mental health service delivery, basic assumptions and philosophy, brief descriptions of what the programs are that one evaluates, and some thoughts about how evaluation relates to accountability and to the evolution of the science of mental health service delivery. Evaluation broadly defined has the potential both for building a science of service delivery and for moving public policy and programs increasingly toward meeting people's needs.

History of Mental Health Programs

A brief historical perspective is useful to understand the state of mental health programs today and their possibilities for the future.

American psychiatry actually began in the community with the development of the first psychiatric service located in a community general hospital by Benjamin Rush in 1765. In colonial and early America what services existed were delivered locally, largely through the almhouses and jails of the day. It was not until the beginning of the nineteenth century that state and private mental hospitals or asylums were created and not until much later in that century that they became large, overcrowded, and custodial. Earlier, especially during the era of moral treatment in the nineteenth century, they were therapeutic institutions with humane programs much akin to the milieu therapy of today. They also had very comparable discharge rates. As they grew larger and were more poorly staffed (a trend frequently associated with the large immigrations of the middle and latter parts of the century), they lost their therapeutic orientation and potential. Thus, while admissions grew, discharges declined. This was an era largely of hospital-based services, far from local communities. However, even then it became clear that those living near the hospital or on major access and transportation routes used the facilities most. One of the major evaluative studies of the day, the 1855 report by Edward Jarvis, entitled "Insanity and Idiocy in Massachusetts: Report of the Commission on Lunacy," clearly documented this phenomenon. Consistent with the needs and views of the times, Jarvis's report was used to evolve further public policy and to move program

3

development toward building more state hospitals. The last part of that century and the early part of the twentieth saw the evolution of various reform movements that had an impact on mental health services. In this area, the work of Dorothea Dix and of Clifford Beers, as citizens evaluating services, brought to public attention the major abuses in mental health services and led to changes including development of citizen participation—itself a major evaluative instrument and force for change.

Slowly, with the advent of this century, ambulatory care began to come into focus, along with the shift in conceptualization and treatment of mental illness initiated by Freud and Meyer. Early in the century so-called psychopathic, or acute, receiving hospitals were opened closer to population bases. In addition to private office practices, there were the beginnings of public outpatient clinics and so-called satellite clinics serving local communities. The child guidance and orthopsychiatry movements of the second and third decades of the century not only fostered the development of these services but also assisted the beginnings of consultation, education, and preventive efforts, especially in schools. Military psychiatry during both world wars discovered and rediscovered the importance of acute treatment near the front lines in an effort to rapidly reintegrate psychiatric casualties back into their usual social networks.

As psychological and socially oriented therapies improved and as mental health training programs and the work force increased, ambulatory services became increasingly possible and important. The introduction of both the phenothiazines in 1955 and later the antidepressants greatly stimulated this development and made the treatment of the major mental illnesses on an outpatient basis increasingly possible. The development of the National Institute of Mental Health during this era had a major impact on the possibilities for services, training, and research in the country.

Related to a national evaluation effort, the report of the Joint Commission on Mental Health and Illness moved toward the enactment of federal legislation in 1963 to initiate a national community mental health centers program. Experience in Peace Corps psychiatry and other developments of preventive approaches, along with later experience in Vista, the Job Corps, and other OEO programs, opened a new aspect of the field and helped stimulate mental health involvement in broader human services programs. The full-scale development of community participation in these programs furthered the evolution towards community-based services and so-called deinstitutionalization. In the latter part of the 1960s and in this decade, community mental health centers, mental health services within neighborhood health centers, community general hospitals, and other human-service agencies have become more common. During this time, state umbrella agencies of the human services or human resources variety with mental health and retardation as integral components have also developed. Despite a split at the national level, the current era has seen a tendency at state and local levels to integrate mental health and retardation services.

As services have developed, attempts have been made to build in program evaluation. This book tells the story of some of those efforts. First, however, it is useful to describe some of the assumptions and program patterns in the field of mental health, as they are the bases for evaluation efforts.

Basic Assumptions and Philosophy

Current programming evolves from clinical and research experience as an attempt to provide for people's service needs. Certain assumptions have evolved which are so built into our thinking that they are rarely examined. They do provide some underpinnings for programs; further evaluation of these as a beginning might contribute to the development of a science of mental health service delivery. While these assumptions might seem very simple and common-sensical, it is nonetheless useful to make them explicit if they are to be useful for generating testable hypotheses. Let us briefly examine some of them, keeping in mind both the historical perspective and the following descriptions of programs.

1. Services should be located close to population centers. It is assumed that accessibility and availability of services, as a part of the community, will ensure maximal utilization. Programs are therefore "decentralized" to local towns, cities, neighborhoods, and areas.

2. Mental health services can be relevant to the life issues of potential consumers. There is an assumption that people define their problems in mental health terms, or that mental health services can be built into other caregiving systems or can be defined in ways which are syntonic with the ways in which consumers define their needs for outside assistance.

3. Comprehensive, continuous services are necessary. It is assumed that patients need and can make use of a variety of services and that continuity of care is essential.

4. Community-based care is preferable to institutionalization wherever possible. It is assumed that it is more useful to treat patients in the context of family, work, and community networks rather than in more distant, isolated facilities, although there is a recognition that both inpatient and a variety of ambulatory services are required.

5. Early case identification and treatment are important for outcome and prevention. It is assumed that chronicity can be prevented and morbidity reduced in this way.

6. The public health model can be applied to mental health. It is assumed that a population-centered perspective can be applied to mental health planning, program development, and implementation and that despite a lack of definitive knowledge regarding etiology, prevention is at least possible. Natural support systems and crisis intervention are thought to be integral aspects of such efforts.

7. Various treatment modalities are effective. It is assumed that a variety of

treatments (provided by a variety of professionals and paraprofessionals) from the psychological through the social and biological do, in fact, affect the natural course of mental illness.

8. Mental health consultation and education are effective. It is assumed that these functions do affect caregivers, consumers, and the population at large in terms of therapeutic, preventive, or mental health promotion efforts. It is further assumed that human psychological development can be fostered and mental health can be enhanced through these techniques related to times of crisis and stress or to the ongoing development of individuals.

9. Mental health and illness are determined by many things. It is assumed that psychological, social, and biological factors are interweaved in this dimension of human existence.

10. Mental health services need citizen input. It is assumed that citizen input—be it advisory, participatory, or controlling—provides useful direction for service delivery.

11. Training and education produce more effective workers. It is assumed, whatever the treatment or preventive modality, that training enhances therapeutic impact.

12. Integrated services are valuable. It is assumed at the service delivery level that the integration of mental health, retardation, and other human services, including education, in most instances is useful and that this speaks to service integration at other organizational levels of government.

13. Mental health services can be cost-effective. It is assumed that services can be efficient, effective, and cost-controlled and that it might be possible to monitor costs and to begin to quantify benefits.

14. Mental health services are best based on need. It is assumed that services can be related to population needs and that there can be such indicators which lead to rational planning.

This brief outline demonstrates both the scope of our assumptions and the major limitations of our current knowledge in this field. It clearly points to the critical need both for evaluation and for the development of a scientific basis for mental health service delivery. In the current absence of such data and evaluation, many of these assumptions have been translated into programs.

Mental Health Programs—Current and Future

While an in-depth description of mental health programs is beyond the scope of this chapter, some of the patterns of service delivery currently employed are briefly outlined here. Also reviewed are some of the future trends. Familiar as these programs are to many readers, they (along with our assumptions) are the bases for our evaluation efforts and are founded upon some of the potentially testable assumptions described previously.

Hospital-based Programs

Public and private hospitals provide a range of diagnostic and treatment services. Increasingly, community general hospitals are developing mental health units in local communities. The large mental hospitals may also serve as sites for partial (day or night care) hospitalization and for outpatient services. Some are beginning to become human-service institutions or campuses providing a range of services. Frequently the hospital serves a defined geographic or population area, and it may have units targeted to specific population bases. Many hospitals are linked to community services which provide before-and-after care.

Community-based Services

Community mental health centers serve defined populations of 50,000 to 200,000. They provide inpatient care, partial hospitalization, outpatient services, emergency care, and consultation and education as essential services. In addition, centers have come to provide specialized diagnostic programs, mental retardation services, linkages to state hospital services, children's services, before-and-after care for state hospital patients, rehabilitation services, community alternatives (halfway houses, cooperative apartments, foster care, etc.), training, research, and evaluation. Community participation is included in both public and private centers. Several patterns have emerged, including both centralized programs and decentralized services operating out of multiple sites in the community. Affiliations with a variety of health, social service, and educational agencies have been made. The most frequent basic model has been the "multiple-agency center" involving at least two participants, a general hospital and a mental health outpatient clinic (each may be publically supported, private, or nonprofit corporations). Many centers have evolved toward decentralized models linked to neighborhood health or multiservice centers as well as other community agencies where staff and programs are integral parts of these other agencies. The latest community mental health center legislation (1975) actually mandates this kind of programming.

Neighborhood psychiatry involves a recent pattern of service delivery that locates mental health services in neighborhood settings. This includes solo neighborhood mental health centers as well as services within comprehensive neighborhood health and human-service centers. It encompasses several models of practice. The first model includes only mental health consultation. The second is a mental health service operating in isolation within a neighborhood health center. A third prototype is that of complete ambulatory mental health service that is fully integrated into the comprehensive health center. A last model is one where mental health services are fully integrated into the center and a mental health professional is in a position of executive responsibility within this comprehensive delivery system.

Mental health services in nonhealth agencies are services that are provided in schools, preschool programs, work, welfare, religious organizations, legal services, prisons, courts, police, colleges, and the like. Both direct and indirect services are provided within these programs of broader purpose. These services have the potential for being relevant to people's needs and to the way in which they define the need for outside assistance.

Mental health consultation and education are so-called indirect services, consisting of case- and consultee-centered consultation, as well as program- and consultee-centered administrative consultation, and various educational approaches including anticipatory guidance, which provide the basis for broad population-centered approaches. Collaboration, coordination, cooperation, and community development and action are newer, less well defined community mental health approaches.

Self-help and support systems are formal and informal networks and groups formed within the community to address problems and issues relevant to people's lives without defining the participants as patients. They are thought to have great potential for prevention and mental health promotion.

Mental health in government agencies is dealt with in programs that include administration as well as the provision of direct and indirect services. These have included work within the military, Peace Corps, OEO, Job Corps, Vista, and various state and local governmental agencies.

Community alternatives to institutionalization are mentioned as part of community mental health center programming. This aspect of so-called deinstitutionalization involves the development of halfway houses, group homes, cooperative apartments, foster homes, and the like, and has become an important aspect of mental health services in the community.

Work and rehabilitation programs of a vocational, habilitative, and rehabilitative nature have increasingly become a crucial aspect of the mental health system.

Comprehensive health and human services involve—at state and local delivery levels—mental health services that have become integrated with such other service systems as mental retardation, public health, welfare, corrections, children's and youth services, family services, and education.

This brief outline of evolving patterns of mental health service delivery and practice, speaking both to current activities and to future directions, is not intended to be exhaustive. It highlights the dimensions of our field and outlines some of the bases for evaluation now and in the foreseeable future. Program planners and developers are attempting to translate clinical and research knowledge and experience into programs that are increasingly relevant to people's needs. This constitutes the art of mental health planning and service delivery.

Evaluation and Accountability: Toward a
Science of Mental Health Service Delivery

We are at a point in the evolution of our services where one needs to be increasingly accountable and where one must move forward in terms of developing a science of mental health service delivery. Many have been concerned about this for a number of years; their concern and interest as scientists are being increasingly bolstered by a need for accountability to a number of different kinds of groups. For example, accountability of mental health service delivery by practitioners and administrators to the government increases year by year in terms of the ways in which funding is developed and the ways in which one has to document what is done along with its productiveness and its cost. This is a major issue in terms of insurance carriers (other than governmental) as well. There is a need to be accountable to ourselves and to the professions that many of us represent. There has been an increased need over the past fifteen years to be accountable to the citizens who, in the long run, provide much of the funding that makes our efforts possible. There is also an increase in recognition of the need to be accountable to patients or consumers. The days are over when we can say: "We know we have done good work." We have considerable experience that will allow us to provide many different kinds of data that will indicate what we have been able to accomplish. There is a much more stringent tone in the country in terms of what people expect, and people are increasingly aware of their right to know what it is that they are buying in time, dollars, and resources. The current mood views mental health as a product of a system. The development of an evaluation system, in a manner that leads to a science of the delivery of services, will make us increasingly accountable and increasingly scientific as well.

There are many other ways in which evaluation is important in terms of the development and implementation of public policy—ways in which such policy evolves and ways in which public policy is translated into programmatic activities. One of the sources of the evolution of new and innovative ideas is program evaluation. This is a beginning in the understanding of what the gaps in services are and what our services actually provide. We must look at where we are effective as well as ineffective and inefficient. This can dictate new directions in terms of public policy, which can be translated into new programs that, when evaluated, can develop a kind of feedback that allows for public policy to change and for programs to change.

Of course, there are many other forces which determine public policy. It is not exclusively dictated by what our research or evaluation or epidemiological approaches indicate are in the best interest of taking care of people. There is a way in which these other dimensions can enhance what formal program evaluation can provide in the development of public policy. There really is a way in which the input of our patients, consumers, and citizens concerning the gaps in our services (whether or not we are providing what they need) is particularly important. It is a kind of informal evaluation, if you will, which many people who have functioned in a public administrative capacity recognize not only as a constant source of pressure but also as a valuable input. This is a kind of program evaluation that has never been formalized and one that needs to be built upon in terms of beginning to understand what people's needs are—as they themselves define those needs. This means that we must move increasingly not only toward delivering services but to delivering them in the most relevant fashion possible to the people who would be our consumers. The political process, of course, refines public policy, and this serves as another source of evaluation. In that sense, politics is not all bad; frequently it is responsive to the needs of people and the ways in which people wish to have their services delivered.

The judicial process is another source of public policy and evaluation. In many states there are law suits, which in a sense are part of an evaluative process, assessing the quality and the gaps in the services that we provide. This, too, can be another feed-in for the determination of public policy. If one looks at evaluation in a broad sense, it must include not only formal program evaluation but also numerous other avenues of scrutiny and feedback. In the development of public policy, program evaluation of these various sorts must feed back into the changing of operations that, hopefully, will be consistent with what people need.

Of course, there is a major problem with resources in the evaluation process. It is striking how little we have in the way of evaluation dollars. The number of positions we have for direct services is always our major emphasis, and recognition has come late that we have to evaluate what these people do. There will be, no doubt, increasing pressure to develop new resources, or perhaps certain kinds of evaluation will become increasingly reimbursable, or we will have to alter our priorities so that we give evaluation increasing emphasis as part of the total delivery system. Evaluation, in that sense, needs to be treated as part of the service function as it feeds back upon operations and increases their efficiency.

The current pressures toward increased accountability add new emphasis to program evaluation even while funds are scarce. We are at a point where various program ideas and treatment modalities can be evaluated, where experiments in nature do exist, where comparative and controlled studies can be accomplished, and where the assumptions we have enumerated can be tested. With adequate safeguards for human rights, community and public knowledge, participation, and scrutiny, we can now develop and use modern evaluation tools. We must have the security and basic self-esteem to allow ourselves and our programs to be evaluated and to change our views and services if they do not stand the test. The field of mental health service delivery can be defined, and it can achieve both theoretical and scientific evaluative underpinnings. Instead of our programs being based upon our good intentions and subject to all the forces of history and current circumstance, they can develop a basis in sound evaluation that will help them to survive over time. Operational and applied research are the cornerstone of these new efforts.

2

The Changing Environment and Purposes of Mental Health Program Evaluation

Herbert C. Schulberg

A review of developments in mental health program evaluation can be approached from various perspectives. The review could document and stress the wide gap still separating present evaluative practices from desirable standards, or it could direct attention to the progress that is occurring despite formidable methodological obstacles and ambivalent organizational mandates. The first vantage point is factually accurate but unduly pessimistic. The second focus is less idealistic but more optimistic and constructive. This overview, therefore, approaches the past and present of program evaluation in the mental health field within the latter framework of what could be called "positive realism."

This framework of positive realism is best clarified by relating mental health program evaluation to: (1) the evolving organizational environments within which it is practiced; (2) the changing concepts and purposes guiding this activity; (3) the improved technologies available to its practitioners; and (4) the growing uses being made of evaluation findings. Since the latter two areas of concern are considered at length in this book's subsequent chapters, this chapter will focus upon the environments and purposes of mental health program evaluation. The time frame to be reviewed is the decade of 1965 to 1975, a period during which the 1963 federal Community Mental Health Centers Act stimulated many of the field's advances.

The Environment of Program Evaluation

Clinicians, administrators, and researchers engaged in program evaluation usually experience distress, even culture shock, as they become familiar with the requirements and nuances of this field. Clinicians and administrators generally react to evaluative studies with ambivalence, if not negativism. They overcome initial resistances by establishing unrealistic expectations of the value of data. Since evaluative findings usually fail to meet these expectations, disillusionment sets in and prior negativism is reinforced. If evaluation is to survive, the clinician and administrator must reconcile presumed needs for evaluative data with the pragmatic realities within which evaluators function. Most significantly, the clinician and administrator must permit assessment methodologies and information-gathering techniques to be advanced within their organizations. Productive

13

environments for program evaluation are created most successfully when all staff members recognize their interdependency in achieving the organization's immediate and long-term goals.

Program evaluators, similarly, have disquieting experiences when first participating in evaluative enterprises. Perhaps the most painful lesson to be learned by fledgling evaluators, particularly if they are sophisticated methodologists, is that the real world within which programs operate and assessment is conducted bears little resemblance to the controlled environment of laboratories. More specifically, evaluators have little control, if any, over the relationships between stimuli and responses; and their research often is subject to the whims of clinical and administrative decisionmakers. Thus, evaluators generally must adapt to the rules and mores of service-oriented environments; these environments rarely adapt to the evaluator's methodological needs!

Implicit in this fundamental premise about the ethos for assessment is the fact that program evaluation concerns itself not with isolated relationships between a specific clinician's therapeutic activities and the patient's subsequent adjustment but, rather, with an organization's broader set of activities (Schulberg, Sheldon and Baker, 1970). These activities occur within a social and technological system; they have specific inputs of resources and conditions, techniques for establishing relations among them, and outputs that can be evaluated against given standards. Additionally, aspects of the organization's patterned activities occur not only within its own structure but in relation to other organizations as well.

Accepting this open-system conception of the mental health program evaluator's work environment, what changes have occurred within it over the past decade? Clearly, the most dramatic alterations stem from markedly heightened expectations of what constitutes comprehensive mental health services. Prior to 1965, few centers or programs provided more than a limited number of services. Inpatient and outpatient care were common, emergency services and partial hospitalization less so, while consultation and education were discussed in classrooms but rarely practiced in the community. The Community Mental Health Centers Act deemed all five of these services as "essential." Furthermore, the Act and its Regulations imposed the additional requirement that essential services be accessible and available and that they afford continuity of care to all persons regardless of age, sex, race, income level, diagnosis, etc. All persons residing in the center's catchment area were to be eligible for clinically indicated services.

The implications of these requirements have been mind-boggling to both administrators and program evaluators. No longer did it suffice for a general hospital to provide exemplary inpatient services if they were unrelated to a patient's preadmission needs and postdischarge follow-up. No longer could the child guidance clinic content itself to perform highly sophisticated diagnostic workups with children of middle-class families while overlooking the needs of children from surrounding lower-class neighborhoods. No longer could researchers be smugly self-satisfied with sophisticated studies of relatively esoteric matters like verbal interaction patterns between patient and therapist while ignoring the question of which patients receive psychotherapy and which drug therapy. No longer could evaluators produce reports emphasizing abstract principles devoid of practical utility.

A list of the environmental alterations produced for the program evaluator by community mental health activities could be extended at length, but it suffices here to emphasize that the evaluator's personal work setting and frame of reference have undergone profound modifications in recent years. Of particular significance is that community mental health evaluators now must devote considerably more attention to the extraorganizational variables affecting patient care and can no longer restrict their focus to intraorganizational factors alone. Schulberg and Baker (1970) have noted that concepts drawn from open-systems theory are particularly helpful to the evaluator in exploring a mental health center's primary task, the nature of its inputs and outputs, environmental conditions, and subsystem interactions. As will be noted shortly, a direct consequence of this change in environmental focus has been a shift in the very purposes for which evaluations are performed.

A full description of the changing environment within which mental health program evaluation occurs must also take note of the growing linkages between community mental health services and the broader human-services field. The past decade's sociopolitical movements have been relevant to community mental health in that they have stimulated wide-ranging efforts to rectify the varied problems besetting America's less fortunate citizens.

Of particular interest is that planners and program directors, for the first time, acknowledged that mentally ill persons have needs that can best be met by caregivers who are not involved in the field of mental health. If an indigent mentally ill person discharged from inpatient care is to adjust successfully in the community, it is essential that he or she receive not only psychiatric follow-up but also the services of public welfare workers, vocational and social rehabilitation therapists, recreational therapists, etc. Clearly, a wide range of human services, rather than only psychiatric ones, are vital to maintaining former patients in community settings.

When planners design broad human-services systems rather than narrow categorical ones, the implications for the program evaluator are multiple. Again, a systems perspective must be utilized to assess the flow of patients into and out of the community mental health program. It becomes even more vital, however, in wide-ranging programs for the clinician and evaluator to identify what services produce what outcomes. For too long, assessment studies have failed to specify the processes whereby, and the time frames during which, therapeutic interventions produce identifiable outcomes. Consequently, far too much program evaluation has pursued data only randomly related to the clinician's expectations of how and when change would occur.

Reaching meaningful conclusions under such circumstances is obviously difficult, if not impossible. After reviewing the limited ability of program evaluation efforts to affect federal policy, Horst (Horst et al. 1974) formulated two propositions about why programs and their evaluations are ineffective: (1) the problem addressed, the intervention being made, and the outcome expected are not sufficiently well defined to be measurable; and (2) assumptions linking expenditure of resources, program interventions, and the immediate outcome to be caused by the interventions are not specified or understood clearly enough to permit their testing.

A decade ago, Freeman and Sherwood (1965) stressed the need for clinicians and researchers to establish an "impact model" which would guide any program's operation and evaluation. The model would include a set of theoretical concepts that trace the dynamics of how the program produces desired effects; i.e., it logically interrelates a set of principles and procedures with desired outcomes. When such a model is available, hypotheses can be tested and outcomes evaluated through valid research procedures. In the absence of such a model, it is all too easy to confuse spurious relationships with the conclusion that the activity under study did indeed produce the hypothesized result. If the context within which mental health programs operate continues to broaden, as is suggested here, impact models will be needed more than ever to assess validly the effectiveness of care provided psychiatric patients within human-services networks.

Purposes of Program Evaluation

As the size and focus of mental health programs have changed over the past decade, shifts inevitably have occurred in strategies for evaluating them. Continued impetus for this evolution will stem from the requirements in Title III of the Health Services and Nurse Training Act of 1975 (PL 94-63) that mental health centers establish ongoing quality-assurance programs, including utilization and peer review systems, respecting the centers' services (Windle and Ochberg, 1975). As a direct consequence of this statute, the purposes of future assessment procedures will include measuring fiscal efficiency, determining adequacy of services relative to community need, and evaluating patient results. These future emphases are markedly different from those of earlier program evaluation ventures, which focused primarily on effort assessments.

A review of these imminent shifts and their implications is best undertaken by considering the relationship between organizational goal achievement and program evaluation. Mental health centers have been pressured during the past decade to function as "self-evaluating organizations," a direction certainly reinforced by PL 94-63. However, Wildavsky (1972) has noted that evaluation and organization may be contradictory terms, since "evaluation" suggests skepticism and is oriented towards change, and "organization" implies stability and generates commitment.

Most organizations evaluate policies and programs only periodically. Self-evaluating organizations do so continuously and must educate staff to tolerate the anxieties produced by constant change. Furthermore, the self-evaluating organization demands problem solving divorced from commitments to specific policies and organizational structures. Cynicism may grow, however, among staff as earlier wisdoms repeatedly are replaced by new truths. This enigma is particularly striking within community mental health centers, since many of their activities are derived from emerging ideologies rather than being founded upon scientific knowledge (Schulberg and Baker, 1969). When operating within an organization required to function in both a contemporary and effective manner, administrators are challenged regularly to "unsell" old policies in favor of new ones that are more in keeping with current fads or mandates, while simultaneously retaining the loyalty of staff whose personal beliefs are constantly being eroded.

Upsetting as these tensions may be within self-evaluating organizations, they, nevertheless force staff to recognize that evaluation is not a task performed in isolation from other administrative functions. Rather, it is integral to a larger sequence of events in the cycle of planned change. James (1962) emphasized this principle many years ago, but mental health centers are still fumbling for ways to routinize the linkages between planning, service operation, and evaluation. Rather than viewing these three responsibilities as related components in an ongoing cycle of program development, too often they are perceived and managed by staff as discrete, separable activities.

Reasons for the poor and tenuous links between evaluation and planning-service operations have been widely reviewed (see Wholey et al. 1970; Rossi and Williams, 1972). In this context of analyzing how evaluative purposes are changing, it is apt to cite Halpert's (1973) conclusion that evaluators and administrators work poorly together because they pay little attention to each other's concerns. Evaluators, pursuing an analytic orientation, are preoccupied with determining researchable questions to be studied through valid methods and techniques. Administrators, preoccupied with service provision, seek answers but pay little heed to the framing of researchable questions. Given these divergent mental sets, it isn't surprising that in many mental health centers, evaluators miss contributions to program development by focusing on questions they deem answerable rather than those that administrators want answered most. Similarly, administrators often forego analytic contributions to program development by failing to frame answerable questions, or by demanding mounds of data irrelevant to their true concerns.

When approached in a spirit of constructive interaction, the questions for which administrators may expect the evaluators' help can be categorized as follows (James 1962; Suchman 1967):[1]

1. Assessment of effort: how are staff utilized and how do these practices compare with local or national standards?
2. Assessment of performance: what outcomes have the program's efforts produced?
3. Assessment of adequacy: to what extent has the community's problem been solved by this program?
4. Assessment of efficiency: can the same outcome be achieved at lower cost?

Each type of question is answered with a different type of data. Administrators, therefore, must specify their information needs with some precision if the evaluator's contribution is to be relevant. A review of present mental health evaluation activities leads to the encouraging conclusion that data needs, indeed, are being expressed in more refined and researchable ways. For example, most administrators now recognize, at least superficially, that they cannot pose global inquiries about their program's worth to evaluators. Instead, questions must relate to whether defined outcome criteria have been achieved under given conditions of resource allocation and service operation. Thus, the repeated admonition in the evaluation literature that program objectives must be specified before assessment can be initiated seems to be paying off.

Concomitant to this sharpening process, there has been a shift in the types of questions being posed to evaluators by administrators and policymakers. The most marked of these information shifts is a decreased concern with how mental health center staff spend their time, and an increased emphasis upon evaluating the product of staff efforts. Hargreaves (Hargreaves et al. 1975) provides an overview of motivations for assessing performance and includes a sampler of twenty-three research instruments available for this purpose. Goal attainment scaling, which differs conceptually from other measurement approaches, provides a further opportunity for determining the effectiveness of therapeutic interventions. The growth of sophisticated management information systems is a particularly welcome development in furthering studies of how staff utilization patterns relate to client outcome (Broskowski, in press). Analyses of outcome, in turn, have propelled questions of cost efficiency to the forefront. Critical questions about program adequacy also have become answerable with the advent of management information systems, and such queries, consequently, are being raised more frequently.

The shifting purposes of evaluation contain direct and indirect implications for mental health policy and program practices. Outcome studies, for years regarded as necessary but unfeasible, now require that clinicians specify patient problems, treatment approaches, and operationally defined results expected at stated periods of time. Thus, in meeting the technical requirements of outcome evaluation, clinicians have been challenged to modify various patient care practices. For example, they have been forced to consider how alternative treatment goals can be achieved effectively in time-specified frameworks, and what the relative costs are of differing treatment approaches to accomplish specified goals.

In present times of fiscal austerity and even budgetary reductions for mental health services, the feasibility of both evaluating treatment outcome and performing cost-efficiency assessments is creating profound anxiety among practitioners long accustomed to viewing such analyses as irrelevant to their work habits. The dearth of valid and reliable outcome studies had legitimated the clinicians' opposition to evaluation pressures, but their resistance is crumbling under the combined weight of legislative demands for fiscal data and improved management information system capability. Cost-benefit and cost-efficiency assessments are sure to receive increased attention during the coming years, and suggestions for their productive use are offered by Rosenthal (1975).

Finally, questions as to whether a mental health center's services are meeting the needs of community residents are also moving to the forefront of evaluative concern. Long a matter of intellectual speculation rather than actual study, adequacy evaluation now is mandated by PL 94-63. Adequacy of center services can be studied from such diverse perspectives as consumer attitudes, epidemiologic findings, or social and demographic profiles (Hargreaves et al. 1974). Regardless of which specific approach is utilized, each requires that adequacy of center services be assessed in relation to community-oriented criteria rather than staff predilections.

When a mental health center indeed functions as a self-evaluating organization, it must constantly ponder the systemic implications of program modifications. The questions and methodologies of evaluation, therefore, should reflect a systems orientation, emphasizing that degree of success in achieving certain organizational objectives must be analyzed in relation to organizational performance on other functions. In contrast to the goal attainment model that would focus evaluative scrutiny on any given clinical activity in isolation from other center programs, the system model of evaluation poses the broader question: In how balanced a manner is the mental health center achieving its multiple purposes? Etzioni (1960) first directed attention to this more global evaluative perspective, and its relevance increases as mental health centers are mandated to provide an expanding array of services.

The system model of evaluation assumes a balanced organizational effort to achieve all goals through an optimal distribution of available resources, not the maximal satisfaction of any one goal to the detriment of others. Determining the relative worth and balance of organizational goals, and assessing whether they have been achieved, involves highly complex judgments, usually rooted in and guided by covert value choices. Since the system's key participants often do not share identical values, Edwards, Guttentag, and Snapper (1975) have asserted that the central need in present evaluative activities is the design of a conceptual framework linking inferences about the state of the world, the decisionmakers' values, and program decisions.[2] Since priorities for evaluating staff effort, patient outcome, cost efficiency, or program adequacy emanate from differing value frameworks, congruence in the value judgments of administrators, clinicians, researchers, and consumers must constantly be strived for if assessment studies are to be undertaken and analyzed from a common vantage point.

Finally, even if value congruence can be achieved among relevant parties, there still remains the need to ascertain that a fit exists between the type of evaluation being performed and the decision that it is intended to affect. Weiss (1974) has ruefully noted that forcing all evaluations into a single mold, particularly that of assessing patient outcome, can have perverse consequences. She therefore distinguishes between evaluations relevant to policy, strategic, or tactical decisions. The policy decision deals with options at the highest legislative or administrative levels, the strategic with choices regarding mode of operation, and the tactical with alternatives in daily program practices. Since the consequences of decisions at each of these levels vary considerably, evaluation procedures should differ commensurately with regard to methodology, data collection, and expense. Policy decisions require prospective social experimentation incorporating maximal scientific rigor. Strategic decisions can utilize evaluation performed under conditions that compromise optimal design requirements, while tactical decisions can benefit from the variety of data routinely reported by sophisticated management information systems.

Summary

Progress in evaluating mental health programs is occurring despite formidable methodological obstacles and ambivalent organizational mandates. This progress is most evident when examining the evolving environments within which evaluation is practiced and the changing concepts and purposes guiding this activity. As community mental health programs have expanded their range of services, evaluators have turned more attention to the extraorganizational factors affecting patient care. Open systems theory is particularly relevant to the assessment of a mental health center's primary task, the nature of its inputs and outputs, environmental conditions, and subsystem interactions.

The expanded environment within which mental health programs operate has produced shifts in the very purposes for which evaluations are performed. There is less concern with how mental health center staff members spend their time and more emphasis upon evaluating the product of staff efforts. Analyses of outcome, in turn, have propelled questions of cost efficiency to the forefront. Concerns about program adequacy are also being addressed with greater frequency, since the advent of management information systems makes such queries more answerable.

Notes

1. Cf. Chapter 6 of this volume.
2. For an illustration of this technique, see Chapter 11 of this book.

References

Broskowski, A. "Management Information Systems for Planning and Evaluation," in H. Schulberg and F. Baker, eds., *Program Evaluation in the Health Fields*, vol. 2. New York: Behavioral Publications, in press.

Edwards, W., Guttentag, M., and Snapper, K. "A Decision-Theoretic Approach to Evaluation Research," in E. Struening and M. Guttentag, eds., *Handbook of Evaluative Research*, vol. 1. Beverly Hills, Calif.: Sage Publications, 1975.

Etzioni, A. "Two Approaches to Organizational Analysis: A Critique and a Suggestion," *Administrative Science Quarterly*, 1960, 5, 257-278.

Freeman, H., and Sherwood, C. "Research in Large Scale Intervention Programs," and *Journal of Social Issues*, 1965, 21, 11-28.

Halpert, H. "Research Utilization, a Problem in Goal Setting: What Is the Question?" *American Journal of Public Health*, 1973, 63, 377-378.

Hargreaves, W., Attkisson, C., Siegel, L., McIntyre, M., and Sorensen, J. *Resource Materials for Community Mental Health Program Evaluation. Part II: Needs Assessment and Planning.* San Francisco: National Institute of Mental Health, 1974.

_____, _____, _____, _____, and _____. *Resource Materials for Community Mental Health Program Evaluation. Part IV: Evaluating the Effectiveness of Services.* San Francisco: National Institute of Mental Health, 1975.

Horst, P., May, J., Scanlon, J., and Wholey, J. "Program Management and the Federal Evaluator," *Public Administration Review*, 1974, 34, 300-308.

James, G. "Evaluation in Public Health Practice," *American Journal of Public Health*, 1962, 52, 1145-1154.

Rosenthal, G. "The Economics of Human Services," in H. Schulberg and F. Baker, eds., *Developments in Human Services*, vol. 2. New York: Behavioral Publications, 1975.

Rossi, P., and Williams, W. *Evaluating Social Programs: Theory, Practice, and Politics.* New York: Seminar Press, 1972.

Schulberg, H., and Baker, F. "Community Mental Health: The Belief System of the 1960s," *Psychiatric Opinion*, April 1969, 6, 14-26.

_____, and _____. "The Caregiving System in Community Mental Health Programs: An Application of Open Systems Theory," *Community Mental Health Journal*, 1970, 6, 437-446.

Schulberg, H., Sheldon, A., and Baker, F. *Program Evaluation in the Health Fields.* New York: Behavioral Publications, 1970.

Suchman, E. *Evaluative Research: Principles and Practice in Public Service and Social Action Programs.* New York: Russell Sage, 1967.

Weiss, C. "Alternative Models of Program Evaluation," *Social Work*, 1974, 19, 675-681.

Wholey, J., Scanlon, J., Duffy, H., Fukomoto, J., and Vogt, L. *Federal Evaluation Policy.* Washington, D.C.: The Urban Institute, 1970.

Wildavsky, A. "The Self-Evaluating Organization," *Public Administration Review*, Sept.-Oct. 1972, 509-520.

Windle, C., and Ochberg, F. "Enhancing Program Evaluation in the Community Mental Health Centers Program," *Evaluation*, 1975, 2, 31-36.

3

Program Evaluation: The Antidisestablishmentarianism Syndrome

Edgar R. Casper

For anyone striving to achieve a goal in a context where relative success or failure is not immediately visible, the question "How well am I doing?" is an obvious and sensible one.

For human-service bureaucracy in general and mental health and retardation programs in particular, the question of program effectiveness seems particularly relevant, and it is surprising that it has taken so long to reach center stage.

Historically, in a country where social philosophy was dominated by the protestant ethic, government provision of or for human services was not originally, and could not be expected to be, a popular cause. The depression era of the 1930s changed all that, and in one sense in a rather surprising way. Pragmatic political response to citizen groups, mustering under various banners representing constituencies of a variety of categorical disabilities, was not surprising. In fact, rational, functional planning, in the then prevailing social and political climate, would have been astounding. But when the first rash of categorical programs failed to yield visibly miraculous results, the cry "Give us more money and we will do a better job!" was heeded uncritically for almost thirty years. One might have expected a more jaundiced eye, much sooner. At any rate, the result of the efforts of the New Deal was massive proliferation of a vast, cumbrous, and fragmented human-service bureaucracy, with different and complex funding streams and ever-increasing doubts about program effectiveness.

Now the pressure is on. More and more program statutes and regulations require, in double time, program evaluation as a condition of funding. There is no problem, obviously, with the basic idea. What is of concern, and what prompts this chapter, is that the way this process is apparently being handled may, in some instances, add new problems, rather than solve existing ones.

The approach in this chapter is impressionistic, and the reader is invited to assess the significance and validity of these observations in the light of her or his vantage point, knowledge, and experience.

In the first place, the relatively sudden and strong pressure in the direction of evaluation appears to be the result of an uneasy political alliance. One group of proponents seems to articulate a genuine desire to promote improvement in the delivery of human services and regards stocktaking, in terms of program evaluation, as a sine qua non toward that end.

23

Another group, on the other hand, seems to place emphasis on "fiscal integrity," with little, if any, regard for human services. This group expects program evaluation to uncover a terrible waste of money, allowing them to demand the drastic cutting of such programs.

Whatever happens, a basic policy confrontation sooner or later appears unavoidable. The present alliance on the evaluation issue tends to postpone this inevitable collision; as an advocate of an effective human-services system, I would rather see confrontation on basic policy issues begin now.

Furthermore, the statutory posture of program evaluation requirements seems to be part of a current trend to demand immediate solutions to insufficiently defined problems. To be sure, there are some programs, such as corrective surgery or the provision of prosthetic devices to physically handicapped persons, that are readily susceptible to simple evaluation techniques. Even in the mental health and mental retardation field, limited-scope programs, such as personal hygiene training, fit into that category. But these are the exceptions rather than the rule.

In terms of modern human-service objectives in general and mental health and retardation program objectives in particular, the emphasis is on comprehensive services that will (1) maximize total functional potential and (2) maintain total functioning at optimum levels.

Meaningful program evaluation entails outcome measurement of services rendered in terms of functional criteria. We are just now witnessing some beginnings in the collection of meaningful data with respect to the provision of existing services.

This is not a technical paper, but a word on relevant data collection and retrieval is in order. Assuming, *arguendo*, that a serviceable set of functional criteria, against which to measure service performance, is available, ex-post-facto evaluation ("How well have we been doing?") is practically impossible, if corresponding functional descriptions of service activities have not been maintained in the past. Evaluation of future service activities in existing programs becomes possible to the extent that functional service data are *first* developed and maintained.

Evaluation is likely to be most profitable where evaluation components are built into the design of future service activities to be performed in new, planned programs or program systems. Consciousness of the evaluation perspective is likely to affect the design of program structures in terms of variables perceived to bear not directly on program effectiveness, but rather on the ease of measuring it. At any rate, a functional, self-renewing data system is an essential prerequisite to meaningful evaluation.

But let us remember our assumption. Where, pray, are the functional criteria presently available for service outcome measurement? And, equally important, where is the field capability to operationalize such criteria, even if they were presently available?

Designers who themselves test their system in the field will readily recognize "bugs" that will send them back to the drawing board for modifications. But when the system is perceived ready for implementation, great reliance will have to be placed on field personnel. This aspect will require considerable "human factors" engineering and personnel training.

One can speculate on the potential rapidity of development of the state of the art. I, for one, am hopeful that much can be done in a relatively short time. But one thing is certain. The tools for the job expected, nay, mandated, to be done are not, so to speak, on the shelf.

This brings us finally to the title of this piece. There is a story of a young couple that felt that their son was a genius and had him tested for a program for specially gifted children. The boy looked at the questions for a while and then wrote: "I can't answer any of these questions, but I can spell antidisestablishmentarianism." Not being able to measure functional service outcome, the service providers, dependent on continued program funding, will, in all likelihood, proceed to measure something else. And, judging by experience, particularly with respect to state plan administration, the powers that be will probably accept such offerings as the best that can at present be realistically expected.

So what is likely to be the result? More gameplaying, at extra cost, with more diversion from direct services or productive planning. And for those not part of or close to the bureaucracy, there will be another distracting illusion that something constructive is being accomplished.

Furthermore, there is the possibility that the present stance on evaluation may have the psychological effect of (1) encouraging, in the short run, the perpetuation of existing programs, which are "perceived," for good or ill, as tried and trusted, and (2) discouraging radical innovation and experimentation in programming. This would be unfortunate. Therapists and counselors frequently do things that work. They may not know what they are doing or what they have done. Even if they think they know, the results may not be replicable. In short, I think it desirable for people to try out new methods and to continue with techniques that work, even if they cannot be explained.

There is no magic in evaluation systems. Even the most sophisticated systems cannot be expected to capture all relevant data or guarantee the infallibility of built-in judgments. For purposes of shaping program policy, reliance on system findings should be tempered with intelligent skepticism. For example, a training center serving retarded, autistic, and disturbed children shifted the emphasis of its therapeutic and training focus from the child alone to the family. Many of the parents, originally reluctant in their involvement, learned to overcome their "fix my child" orientation and joined the staff in growing enthusiasm for the process and the results of the new approach. At the same time, the center has been experimenting with a recently designed evaluation system that yielded as one of its findings that children treated alone tended to progress faster than children treated with their parents. Did this automatically dictate a reverse shift in therapeutic focus? The center did not think so, and I agree. Reexamination of the system as well as the program is in order before any definitive conclusions can be drawn.

Let us then proceed with developing and refining methods of program planning and evaluation. But let us beware of imposing unrealistic requirements that, by forcing maladaption and fostering illusions, may retard, rather than advance, the cause of improved services. A shift in legislative orientation from pragmatic and fragmented response to lobby group demands to one indicating sensitivity to program coherence and comprehensiveness is to be applauded, but in demanding promptly what cannot be promptly delivered—meaningful program evaluation—legislative haste may be the thief of time.

4

The Three Faces of Evaluation: Policy, Program, and the Public

Carol H. Weiss

Evaluation can contribute to policymaking and the administration of programs, and it can provide evidence for program accountability to constituents and the publics. All these are significant functions, and those of us in the business of evaluation have a tendency to tout them all and justify our efforts on multiple grounds. Evaluation, after all, provides evidence—and if it is done well, objective, dispassionate, persuasive evidence—that can be used as the basis for a variety of decisions. But it has become clear in the history of evaluation experience that the all-purpose evaluation is a rarity, and that we had better know at the outset which set of purposes it is to serve. Then we can begin to develop an evaluation model, system, or study that serves the purposes of policy, of administration and management, of program practice, or of accountability.

What kinds of decisions are we facing in the fields of human services? Certainly there are policy questions: Which new initiatives should be undertaken? Which existing programs should be expanded, institutionalized, modified, or terminated? How should we allocate resources among such components as outreach, prevention, treatment, education, follow-up, and research, and how shall we allocate resources across institutions and agencies?

The administrative questions are equally compelling. What strategies of program operation shall be selected? What techniques shall be emphasized, which staffing patterns, organizational structures, management and planning tools, and reward systems? How can we improve the effectiveness of the agency's operation day to day, month to month?

There is a further set of questions for which evaluation can contribute evidence. There is a set of questions about clients' expectations and goals and how well these are being met. Just as we can press evaluation into service of accountability to the Office of Management and Budget and the Congress, to the Department of Health, Education and Welfare or the State of New York, to community groups and taxpayers, so can we use evaluation to take a consumer's view of effectiveness of programs.[1] Evaluation can serve as a mechanism of accountability for a variety of constituents.

The primary purpose of evaluation is utilitarian. It can serve other functions as well (such as testing theory), but its basic function is to provide evidence about program effectiveness so that wise decisions can be made about the program in the future. But which decisions are we attending to? If we tackle a

27

policy question—e.g., should a particular type of drug abuse program be supported—we need a certain type of evaluation design, data, and analysis. We need to know the effects of the program on persons exposed to the program and randomly assigned controls not exposed; we need outcome data on the extent of drug use among both groups over appropriate intervals of time, and (if for any reason our randomized experimental design were compromised in execution) we need to introduce further procedures to ensure that observed effects are attributable to the program and not to extraneous conditions. With this type of evaluation, we can give to policymakers good information on the extent to which the program is successful in reducing drug abuse, and (depending upon some value criteria about how much success is "enough") we can contribute to decisions about whether to extend, modify, or discontinue the program.

But what can we tell the administrators? Let us assume that the evaluation shows a modest level of success. The program administrators run a particular operation. They want to know how they can improve the services they manage. Which particular techniques of administration and treatment worked well? Which methods should be emphasized and which should be changed or dropped? On which kinds of people were different techniques more or less successful: Did males react differently from females, were older people different from younger, were there differences if people had higher educational levels or received continuity of service from the same worker? What characteristics, actions, and attitudes of staff differentiated those who were successful from those with less effective records? An evaluation dedicated to administrative and practical ends has to have something to say about issues like these.[2]

It is possible for evaluations to be designed with the requisite sophistication to aid both administrators and staff members. Research procedures to tackle them simultaneously are well known, and in fact, most evaluation studies and evaluation systems tend to undertake all this—and more. But in trying to be all things to all people, they almost inevitably run into three serious problems.

1. The overall policy question involves big decisions and the expenditure of large sums. Therefore, decisions should be based on the best and most valid data to be had. Is the program working or isn't it? Is it better than no program at all or better than the kinds of programs traditionally available? Is success (or failure) attributable to the program itself or to outside or transient conditions? To get valid answers to these questions, experimental design with random assignment is required. But under the conditions that fit administrative operations, random assignment is often sacrificed on the altar of operational practicability.[3]

2. A second serious problem in trying to combine the policy and the administrative evaluation is that, for policy purposes, the program should be explicitly defined and firmly controlled. The policymaker should know precisely what it is that works or does not work. If the program proves good, he or she should know specifically what to fund and set up and have people trained to do.

Those ingredients of the total package that are essential for success should be defined. But again, under most field conditions, when administrators are seeking practical answers to practical questions, the program stimulus is imprecise. It depends on the inevitable vagaries of staffing, organization, structure, the time and the place, the clientele, and the shifts and haphazard changes that occur as outside conditions alter. If the evaluation shows that the program had little success, should the policymaker conclude that programs of this ilk should be abandoned, or is the absence of effect a consequence of specific (and alterable) current conditions?

3. A third problem is the issue of the scale of evaluation—scope and cost. Policymakers (particularly at federal levels but at state levels too) want generalizations: Program A has this much effect across a range of conditions and Program B has that much effect. They need evaluative data across time and place, evaluative evidence that washes out the influence of idiosyncratic personalities and events. On the other hand, the local administrator is concerned about the local program, here and now, and the people it serves. Administrators are not necessarily agog with pleasure at collecting data comparable with that of thirty other programs when the data do not seem germane to the issues at hand. They want to take into account those very local idiosyncracies that seem distorting and misleading to the high-level policymaker.

These are important differences in perspective. The solution, it seems to me, is to gear evaluation designs specifically to the decisions that are going to be made. What decisions are pending? If they are policy decisions (e.g., whether to extend a pilot program to other sites) or if they are administrative decisions (e.g., whether to reduce case loads or use paraprofessionals), the evaluator should select the appropriate questions, criteria, study design, data, and priorities. Only when the key decisions are known can evaluation be planned to yield maximum payoff.[4]

The ideal conditions for evaluation for policy purposes are not easy to come by. We have suggested what the ideal requirements would be: experimental design, an explicit and stable program, and sufficient sites for generalization. These research conditions will yield valid conclusions about program outcomes, and when policymakers are considering allocations in the tens and hundreds of millions of dollars, they should be able to base them on thoroughly credible, valid information. But ongoing programs are not usually hospitable to such research requirements. The imperatives of service—helping people—tend to get in the way.[5]

The closest that researchers have come to ideal policy evaluation is through recent "social experiments." Researchers have undertaken a set of studies geared to developing future programs, such as the negative income tax, housing allowances, and health insurance experiments.[a]

---

[a]The negative income tax and health insurance experiments were begun under the auspices of OEO. HUD is funding the housing allowance experiments, and HEW is running field tests of health maintenance organizations and voucher systems for education.

These "social experiments" are a way of planning rationally for the future. Unlike the backward stance of most evaluative efforts that survey the success of past programming, social experiments involve launching and testing prototypes of new ventures. Their function is to inform the policymaker of the viability and effectiveness of innovations *before* large amounts of money, time, and effort are committed to a major national undertaking. Certainly the last decade has demonstrated that many program ideas that sound persuasive and even unimpeachable in principle. given our present state of knowledge, do not work in operation. If policymakers can look at the consequences of a test run of a program before going "gung-ho" on a nationwide basis, they have the opportunity to reject the ineffective, improve the marginally effective, and mitigate the counterproductive side effects of new programs. It is for this type of major new policy decision that social experimentation is designed.

Social experiments are research. Their goal is to test. They are true experiments, with random assignment of participants to program and. control conditions, and with before and after measurement; the program is explicitly defined and firmly controlled, with the evaluation researchers responsible for ensuring that the program "stimulus" adheres to the prescribed principles and modes of operation. Social experiments tend to be run in several sites with different external environments so that outcomes can be generalized over a range of conditions. Furthermore, if several variants of the basic program are run simultaneously, it is possible to gauge the effects of variations in treatment.

Some social experiments have been run specifically to test possible adverse effects that critics of the proposal have raised. The New Jersey negative-income-tax experiment, for example, was aimed at the question of whether people earning a notch above the guaranteed income would drop out of the labor force. This is a real concern. If there is a substantial drop in work and many more people become eligible for benefits, the program would be much more expensive than advocates claim. So experimentation can produce evidence about negative counterclaims as well as hypothesized benefits of new social programs.

So long as social experiments were more a dream of beleaguered evaluators than a practical reality, there was a tendency to emphasize the advantages and ignore possible limitations.[6] The advantages, if all goes well, are delightful. With this kind of design, evaluation researchers can draw firm conclusions about the merit of a program. Among other things, when the program adheres to well-defined principles and procedures, there is little uncertainty about whether the program has had a fair test or whether its failings are the result of faulty administration or operation. It is probably no accident that most of the new social experiments—the negative income tax, housing allowances, and the health insurance experiments—all involve direct payment of money. Money is easier to control than are services, and it is not subject to the varieties and whimsicalities of human differences.[7]

The recent experience has highlighted some of the difficulties as well. Social experiments are costly,[8] because a prototype program as well as a sophisticated research study has to be administered. Usually it is possible to sample only a few sites, with a sacrifice in generalizability to other places and conditions. When the effects on small scattered groups of recipients are studied, the data may not be representative of outcomes that would have ensued if the program had saturated the areas. Furthermore, even when the researchers are in charge, program operations are not always well handled: external conditions do change, and there are ethical problems in protecting privacy, in obtaining genuine and informed consent from participants, and in giving benefits to an experimental group (and not to controls) and then taking them away after the study is over. Long periods of time can elapse before the results become available for decision purposes, and the reformist impetus that launched the experiment may have dwindled. And as with all research, the results may show small and ambiguous differences among groups, so that interpretation is not easy or clear-cut.[9]

Another limitation may be a dearth of plausible new programs to test. Before a social experiment is launched, the hard rational analysis that leads to the development of a new program has to be done: the nature of the social program analyzed, its dynamics explored, the casual linkages hypothesized (or, better yet, understood), effective points of intervention identified, the likelihood of successful intervention plausibly established, the political context for supporting and sustaining the intervention examined and found appropriate, and the likely benefits and the distribution of those benefits deemed sufficient to warrant the social cost. Social experimentation is useful for policymaking only when such analysis has generated a program or policy that is worth the testing. When a new social initiative has been developed and has attained sufficient credibility to be considered by policymakers, social experimentation provides an elegant data base for decisionmaking. The kinds of information that it produces can prevent costly national failures and lead to better informed and more successful choices at the policy level.

Social experiments look toward future plans. But what about policy decisions regarding existing programs? How can we design evaluations that give good measures of the impact of ongoing programs so that policy decisions can be made about expansion, modification, or termination? If good social experimentation is hard when researchers are in control, how can we hope to get valid measures of outcome within the turbulent conditions, pushes, pulls, and political pressures of a working program?

It seems to me that there are two answers. First, when major policy questions are for real, when authentic allocation decisions will hinge on evaluative evidence, the evaluators have to be given the conditions and the control to do the best possible research. Otherwise, they run the danger of producing inadequate or misleading evidence that contributes little to rationality in decisionmaking. This will mean shifting the locus of authority over certain program decisions to the evaluation team.

The second solution is to recognize that go/no-go kinds of policy decisions are relatively rare.[10] On only a few occasions do policymakers truly consider wiping out an ongoing program—even then, it is not usually on the grounds of effectiveness or ineffectiveness.[11] Most programs build up layers of alliances among legislators, bureaucrats, professional guilds, constituents, and publics that protect them from drastic dismemberment. And even in the last few years, when the administration has proposed chopping out a number of major programs, the rationale has been based less on grounds of ineffectiveness than on differences in political philosophy. Evaluations of some programs, like federal grants to low-income college students, found highly successful outcomes and the programs were still scheduled for the axe—because the administration favored loans and work rather than outright subsidies to students.[12]

The policy questions are circumscribed more often than they are posed. Policymakers may ask "Is this program worth continuing?" But even if results should show out-and-out failure, the usual reaction is to patch it up and try again. And most results are not unremittingly bleak. Evaluations often come up with mixed results—some good, some qualified, some poor outcomes—and the appropriate action is to look for modifications in strategy and practice. Thus, what started out as evaluation for policy purposes comes pretty close to evaluation for administrative purposes.

For administrative purposes, traditional evaluation methods—well executed—have considerable potential. By "traditional evaluation" I mean before-after (or before-during-after) evaluation of the effects of ongoing programs under conditions that are usually less than the research ideal. A number of books have been written on methods of conducting good evaluation even under adverse circumstances, and for administrative decisions, even compromise designs can make significant contributions.[13] Usually the service imperatives of ongoing programs preclude randomized assignment to experimental and control groups, and a weak approximation, such as "contrast groups," is resorted to. Further, the program is not under the evaluator's control, so that the stimulus wobbles around in response to internal and external opportunities and constraints. Traditional evaluation, if it is conducted with rigor and sophistication (and some luck), can give good estimates of overall program effectiveness. But given the constraints under which it often operates, it is better suited for comparing the worth of alternative program strategies.[14] Comparative study of the effects of different program components with different populations can yield evidence of what strategies work best with what groups. Variations in mode of operation and intensity of service can be tested as well. When administrators and managers face decisions about whether to emphasize one set of methods or another, to scrap one technique and adopt a different one, the findings of traditional evaluation provide relevant information.[15] By comparing the outcomes of variant approaches and program components within the context of the programs about which decisions will be made, evaluation demonstrates their relative worth in the operating context and helps the decisionmaker choose wisely. Since evaluation takes time and money, this approach is not likely to be worthwhile for assessing minor program features, but when choices of some magnitude are contemplated, it can make a significant contribution to the rationality of decisionmaking.

There is a further development that can have important impact. One of the pervasive problems with many past evaluations has been that they have been one-shot affairs. The evaluators come in, do a study of more or less elegance, and, after their work is over, depart. But what about the rest of the time? Decisions still have to be made on a regular basis on all kinds of matters—intake criteria, staffing, hours of service, and so on. To meet continuing needs for decisionmaking, evaluative data can be built into an ongoing information system.[16]

Most programs collect data, in fact often vast quantities of data, on clients, staff, finances, process, and plans. With the available computer technology, what used to be file cards in file boxes are now more likely to be computer files. Within the past decade, much effort has gone into turning the scattered bits and pieces of information, originally collected for a variety of different reasons, into comprehensive data systems for management use. But not many of the systems have included evaluative data—data on client outcomes—as part of the array. Sometimes these data are not very hard to include. Even without the paraphernalia of computers, relatively simple measures of program success can be devised (e.g., job placement, maintenance of one's own home) and follow-up data collected on a systematic basis.[b] With this input, the information system has the capability for analyzing a wide range of program conditions (e.g., length of service, referral flow, unit costs) versus the types of client outcomes that ensued. If the data are selected and arranged with due care, such information can provide enormously useful guidance for decisionmaking on a regular basis.

However, one thing we have learned is that program managers are likely to need some training in how to best make use of such information, at both the input and output end.[17] At the input end, they have to be involved in defining what data go into the system—what data are important. One reason that even sophisticated information systems have often been neglected is data overload. Too much information is spewed out—more than decisionmakers want, need, or can digest—and much of it is marginal to their concerns. The first essential, then, is that at the outset we need to know the values and priorities of the intended user audience: What program objectives do they most value? On what basis will they judge the merit of the program? Are they concerned only with the achievement of the official goals of the program, or are they also interested in some of the political and symbolic functions that programs serve—degree of effort, style of service, visibility, consumer representation, etc.? By finding out in advance the needs and priorities of the intended users of the data, the information system starts out with two advantages: (1) it knows what informa-

---

[b]For further information on some uses of outcome measures, see Chapters 8 and 9.

tion is valued and therefore likely to be used, and (2) instead of adding more data on top, it can winnow out the unnecessary in advance and concentrate on priorities.[18]

A system like this can be expanded to serve an accountability function. A program is responsible to different publics—to the funders, whether public or private, who provide the money; to its clients who are entitled to effective service; to other organizations, which refer clients, provide collateral services, receive its departing successes or failures; to citizen groups. If information on their image of program goals and priorities is also collected, we can add their concerns into the system.

Once the relevant audiences are identified and their criteria of program effectiveness understood, the evaluator can develop measures of these criteria and put them into the system.[19] Then, at regular intervals, data are produced that display the success of the program on these measures. Since different user audiences are likely to have different programmatic values and priorities, the information system can become multidimensional and produce data that show "success" on the range of different criteria being applied. It may be that there are trade-offs among different criteria, that, for example, one group's criterion of success is inconsistent with a criterion of another group—increased coverage of the target population may be inversely related to client satisfaction with services for example. Data, particularly the trend data over time that such a system produces, highlight such issues and may help lead to their resolution.

With the outcome data defined by the relevant user groups, the accountability system allows periodic reporting to each group of how well the program is doing in the group's own terms. The key characteristic of the system is that it provides the information that the audience has defined as relevant to its goals and needs. It enables each group to make decisions and take actions on the basis of the kind of information that it values.

It is important to keep the basic system as simple as possible so that the data clearly show what each audience wants to know. Furthermore, most users will need help in interpreting the data and understanding the implications of the data for action. This kind of educational and interpretive input is an important part of any information system.

There should also be incentives and rewards for putting evaluation findings to use. This is a big subject in itself and deserves more than passing mention.[20] But here, let me note, it is possible that one way to motivate decisionmakers to pay attention to evaluation data is to report findings to an array of actors—administrators, practitioners, clients, program planners, funders—and to trust in a legal kind of adversary proceeding to provide incentives for action. Each user group is encouraged to work for changes that will improve performance on the criteria that they have set, and each user group has a way of checking on the progress that is made.

This is the rosy picture. As in earlier days, when social experiments were expected to lead to dramatic advances, the early "advocacy" days of account-ability also promise grand effects. But the result of reporting evaluative data to a wide range of actors can be to politicize the program and can lead to conflict. Murphy and Cohen in their report on "Accountability in Education—The Michigan Experience" describe a situation where the state board of education released evaluative data to legislators, school boards, superintendents, teachers, and parents.[21] As a result of the barrage of criticism that ensued, the entire evaluation program was revised in the second year, and revised again in the third, so that the original intent of distinguishing effective from ineffective schooling was abandoned. Accountability may be able to stimulate action, as its advocates contend, and it has persuasive elements of logic and equity on its side. But we still have much to learn about ways of reaping the constructive contributions and avoiding the controversies and conflicts it can engender. The incentives for improving performance that are allegedly supplied by putting knowledge in the hands of "countervailing actors" are, at the least, double-edged.

One of the things an evaluator always asks of a program before undertaking a study is "What are the goals?" It is a question we less often ask about evaluation itself. But if we had to answer the question, the primary answer would be that evaluation should make for better human services and wiser allocation of resources among and within programs. I have suggested that the goal is best accomplished by adapting the style and content of evaluation research to the needs of those who will use the findings. There always have been, and perhaps always will be, constraints on our ability to fit the knowledge to the need. Barriers of evaluation methodology, difficulty in interpreting ambiguous results, and political pressures that bound the decisionmaking environment may be eternal complaints in the evaluation literature.[22] But if the obstacles to the best of all possible evaluations cannot be removed, they can be navigated. Our record has not been spectacular so far, but there are enough successes to prove that it can be done. As we design evaluations to fit the needs of decisionmakers—the issues they face, the information that will clarify the issues, and the salience to them of different kinds of information—we stand a better chance of making evaluation genuinely useful.

Notes

1. One of the rare discussions of the consumer's interest in evaluation is D. Caputo, "The Citizen Component of Policy Evaluation," *Policy Studies Journal* 1973, 2:92-97.

2. A similar distinction is made between goal achievement models of evaluation, which focus on global issues and systems or process models, which focus on ongoing program issues. A. Etzioni and E.W. Lehman, "Some Dangers in 'Valid' Social Measurement," *Annals of the American Academy of Political and Social Science*, 1967, 373:1-15.

3. An interesting debate of the pros and cons of experimental design in evaluation is found in R. Weiss and M. Rein, "The Evaluation of Broad-Aim Programs: A Cautionary Case and a Moral," *Administrative Science Quarterly*, 1970, 15:97-109; and in D. Campbell, "Considering the Case against Experimental Evaluations of Social Innovations," *Administrative Science Quarterly*, 1970, 15:110-113.

4. This point is also emphasized in D. Stufflebeam, *Educational Evaluation and Decision Making*. Itasca, Ill.: F.E. Peacock Publishers, 1971.

5. In fact, the conflict is so pervasive that some evaluators have advocated the abandonment of the experimental ideal. They suggest its rigidity causes more difficulties than it is worth. See P. Marris and M. Rein, *Dilemmas of Social Reform*. New York: Atherton Press, 1969. Also see E. Guba and D. Stufflebeam, "Evaluation: The Process of Stimulating, Aiding, and Abetting Insightful Activity," address delivered at the Second National Symposium for Professors of Educational Research, Columbus, Ohio: Evaluation Center, College of Education, Ohio State University. Some critics have even advocated the abandonment of the social science paradigm for evaluation. R. Wolf, in "The Application of Select Legal Concepts to Evaluation," Ph.D. dissertation, University of Illinois at Urbana-Champaign, presents an evaluation paradigm based on legal concepts such as impartial juries and rules of procedure and evidence.

6. For example, Rivlin stated in 1971 that social experiments are the only way to get the information necessary to improve the effectiveness of social services. (A. Rivlin, *Systematic Thinking for Social Action*. Washington, D.C.: Brookings Institute, 1971.) Two years later she noted that there are serious dilemmas—both internal to the design and external in the social context—that make social experimentation "exceedingly tricky," difficult to implement, and potentially damaging to participants. (A. Rivlin, "Social Experiments: The Promises and the Problems," *Evaluation*, 1973, 1:77-78.)

7. An economist has suggested that present evaluation techniques are not appropriate to the assessment of the complex benefits of human service programs. He claims that evaluation research methods are doomed to be at least partly inaccurate when dealing with programs providing collective goods because even the quantity of output (much less the quality) cannot be measured accurately. See M. Olson, "Public Service on the Assembly Line," *Evaluation*, 1973, 1:37-41.

8. "Such an experiment is probably the single most expensive way to gain knowledge." H. Orlans, *Contracting for Knowledge*. Washington, D.C.: Jossey-Bass, 1973, p. 113.

9. For a sober view of the New Jersey negative income tax results by authors who took part in its initial planning, see B.S. Mahoney and W.M. Mahoney, "The New Jersey Negative Income Tax Experiment," paper presented at Brookings conference on social experimentation, 1974.

10. An obvious exception is the pilot program with a built-in cutoff date, for

example the project of changing attitudes toward mental health described by E. Cumming and J. Cumming, *Closed Ranks: Study of Mental Health Education.* Cambridge, Mass.: Harvard University Press, 1957.

11. P. Rossi, "Practice, Method, and Theory in Evaluating Social Action Programs," in *On Fighting Poverty: Perspectives from Experience*, J.L. Sundquist (ed.). New York: Basic Books, 1969, pp. 217-234.

12. N. Friedman and J. Thompson, "The Federal Educational Opportunity Grant Program, a Status Report: Fiscal Year 1970." Report to the U.S. Office of Education. New York: Columbia University, BASR.

13. C.H. Weiss, *Evaluating Action Programs.* Boston: Allyn and Bacon, 1972; C.H. Weiss, *Evaluation Research.* Englewood Cliffs, N.J.: Prentice-Hall Publishing Co., 1972. E. Suchman, *Evaluative Research.* New York: Russell Sage, 1967. W. Williams and P. Rossi, *Evaluating Social Programs: Theory, Practice and Politics.* New York: Seminar Press, 1972.

14. A good example of this strategy of evaluation is J. Vanecko, *Community Action Program Goals for Institutional Change.* Chicago: Center for Urban Studies, University of Illinois, 1969.

15. W. Bateman, in "Assessing Program Effectiveness: A Rating System for Identifying Relative Project Success," *Welfare in Review*, 1968, 6:1-10, recognizes that overall program evaluations can mask differences in effectiveness among individual projects within the same program. Information on relative project effectiveness can be useful for both policy and administration.

16. This may be the most productive function of evaluation research to the program administrators; see E. Suchman, "Action for What?: A Critique of Evaluative Research," in *Evaluating Action Programs*, C. Weiss (ed.). Boston: Allyn and Bacon, 1972. But there are organizational obstacles to overcome before evaluative feedback can be utilized, as is noted in S. Sadofsky, "Utilization of Evaluation Results: Feedback into the Action Program," in *Learning in Action*, J.L. Shmelzer (ed.). Washington, D.C.: Government Printing Office, 1966.

17. Program managers, and organizations generally, frequently need technical help and perspective in understanding the information and advice supplied by evaluation; see A. Downs, "Some Thoughts on Giving People Economic Advice," *American Behavioral Scientist*, 1965, 9:30-32.

18. M. Guttentag, in "Subjectivity and Its Use in Evaluation Research," *Evaluation*, 1973, 1:60-65, suggests that values be quantified in order to use mathematical decision theory models to guide program use of research data.

19. That good measurement requires careful conceptualization and methodological expertise is noted by, among others, R. Levine, "Evaluating the War on Poverty," in *On Fighting Poverty*, J.L. Sundquist (ed.). New York: Basic Books, 1969; and T. Glennan, *Evaluating Federal Manpower Programs: Notes and Observation.* Santa Monica, Calif.: Rand Corporation, 1969; and C.H. Weiss, *Evaluation Research.* Englewood Cliffs, N.J.: Prentice-Hall Publishing Co., 1972.

20. For more than passing mention, see R. Havelock, *Planning for Innovation through Dissemination and Utilization of Knowledge.* Ann Arbor, Mich.: Institute for Social Research, University of Michigan, 1969; C. Weiss, "Utilization of Evaluation: Toward Comparative Study," in House Government Operations Committee, *The Use of Social Research in Federal Domestic Programs*, vol. 3, Washington, D.C.: Government Printing Office, 1967; E. Glaser and H.L. Ross, *Increasing the Utilization of Applied Research Results.* Los Angeles: Human Interaction Research Institute, 1971.

21. J. Murphy and D. Cohen, "Accountability in Education—the Michigan Experience," *The Public Interest*, 1974, 36:53-82.

22. C.H. Weiss, "Where Politics and Evaluation Research Meet," *Evaluation*, 1973, 1:37-45; D.K. Cohen, "Politics and Research: Evaluation of Social Action Programs in Education," in *Evaluating Action Programs*, C.H. Weiss (ed.). Boston: Allyn and Bacon, 1972.

Part II:
Problems and Approaches
in Evaluation

5

Developing Information Systems to Facilitate Quality Assessment in Mental Health

Gary L. Tischler

During the past decade and one half, there has been considerable interchange among investigators from behavioral sciences, social sciences, and public health concerning concepts and methods relevant in assessing the quality of mental health services (Roberts, Greenfield, and Miller 1968; Schulberg, Sheldon, and Baker 1969; Zusman and Ross 1969; Fox and Rappaport 1972; Tischler and Myers 1974). The tempo of the interchanges has increased as a result of a growing demand for accountability on the part of funding sources, third-party payers, consumers, and the body politic, as well as advances in computer technology and instrumentation. These latter advances ensure greater standardization and, therefore, comparability of those data felt necessary for quality appraisal. They include the following:

1. The development of standardized forms for recording data pertinent to the psychiatric evaluation (Katz and Lyerly 1963; Lippman et al. 1969; Raskin et al. 1969; Laska, Simpson, and Bank 1969; Slettin et al. 1970; Spitzer and Endicott 1971).

2. Experimentation with alternative ways of structuring the medical record, particularly the problem-oriented format (Hurst and Walker 1972; Grant and Maletzky 1972; Hayes-Roth, Longabaugh, and Ryback 1972; Ryback and Gardner 1973; Lipp 1973; Novello 1973).

3. The development of scales for measuring mental status and social role performance (Lorr and Klett 1967; DeRogatis, Lipman, and Cove 1973; Evenson et al. 1973; Weissman 1975).

4. Methods for increasing the reliability of psychiatric diagnoses (Robins and Guze 1970; Astrachan et al. 1972; Feighner et al. 1972; Spitzer et al. 1974).

5. The development of computer-based recording, storage, and retrieval systems, as well as methods for their linkage to additional data sources (Eiduson, Brooks, and Motto 1966; Laska, Simpson, and Bank 1967; Baldwin 1972; Evenson et al. 1974; Crawford, Morgan, and Gianturco 1974). These advances in instrumentation and computer technology have, in turn, catalyzed the development of more systematic mechanisms to facilitate process evaluation through the use of criteria-oriented approaches.

Criteria-oriented approaches define quality as a function of the degree to which service provided conforms with established standards of excellence within the field. The assumption underlying this form of evaluation is that persons

41

responsible for organizing and managing service systems can generally agree upon what constitutes high-quality treatment without continually monitoring outcome. According to Donabedian's (1966) usage, criteria may be either normative or empirical. Normative criteria are formulated on the basis of professional opinion around an ideal of what represents excellence in practice. A number of methods have been used to develop such criteria, including: the judgment of highly qualified practitioners (Morehead 1967), textbooks and standard publications (Lembke 1956), panels of experts (Payne 1968; Riedel et al. 1971), and polls of practitioners (Lee and Jones 1933; Mikelbank 1966). Empirical criteria are formulated on the basis of actual patterns of care, as shown by statistical analysis (Brauer 1974). They can be used to compare care in one setting with that in another, or with statistical averages obtained from a number of similar settings.

Over the past decade, several forms of peer review have been conceived that emphasize the utilitarian aspects of applying criteria-oriented approaches to monitoring the quality of medical care (Lembke 1967; Morehead 1967; Kessner, Kalk, and Singer 1973). Richardson (1972a) recognized that traditional methods of peer review were hampered by personal biases of experts. While his attempt to reduce discrepancies in judgments through the use of preestablished sets of standards was successful to some extent, continued experiments shed doubt about the reliability and validity of such criteria (Richardson 1972b). More investigations are needed to achieve this ideal, not only in a medical setting but in a psychiatric one as well. Indeed, the application of criteria-oriented approaches to patient care evaluation in mental health settings has only occurred recently (Richman and Pinsker 1973; Zusman and Slawson 1972; Tischler and Riedel 1973; Goldblatt et al. 1973; Henisz et al. 1974; Miller et al. 1974). The December 1974 issue of the *American Journal of Psychiatry* contains a special section on peer review, including some reports from the private sectors and others from statewide programs. Of these, only the Ohio system (Miller et al. 1974) has developed "patient care criteria packages" and has made maximum use of a computerized data base.

Interestingly, the bulk of the activities noted have primarily addressed issues concerning the delivery of patient care services to a general psychiatric population. Consultative and child care services, two major areas of community mental health center activity, have escaped careful scrutiny. As a result, the development and application of systematic mechanisms for quality appraisal in these two areas is largely absent.

Several theoretical models of community mental health consultation have been proposed (Newton and Levinson 1973; Signell and Scott 1971; Deloughery, Gebbie, and Neuman 1971; Caplan 1970; Rogowski 1968). Efforts have been undertaken to classify: consultees; presenting problems (Caplan 1963; Norman and Forti 1972); consultee-consultant relationships; and consultant role or task functioning (Caplan 1963; Shore and Mannino 1969; Brockbank 1968;

Sanders 1969; Rosenblum 1970; Grosser 1969). Preliminary work on criteria development has taken place (Norman and Forti 1972). The objective assessment of the impact of consultative programs, nevertheless, remains problematic (Weiss 1972; Stephenson 1973). While procedures exist for gathering systematic information on various aspects of the consultative process, an information system suitable for professional review of such activities remains to be developed.

A similar problem exists in relation to child care services. The Multi-State Information System has begun to develop a data base suitable for reviewing clinical services to children. By combining newly developed children's admission and termination forms with already existing forms that record services rendered, a procedure for appraising selected sociodemographic characteristics—presenting problems, sources of referral, service utilization patterns, disposition, and subsequent referral and status upon termination—is available. Recent versions of the admissions and termination forms, however, seem most appropriate for administrative audiences, but have limited utility in relation to quality assessment through criteria-oriented, goal attainment, or multidimensional outcome approaches.

Work in progress at the Pittsburgh Child Guidance Center (Henderson et al. 1972) has focused on developing a data base designed to monitor and serve as an aid in clinical decisionmaking. The system is designed to arrive at treatment, not diagnostic decisions; therefore, data collection is limited to informational items deemed necessary and sufficient for making treatment decisions. This emphasis on minimal data fosters a more rigorous determination of whether information adds predictive power or contributes to more accurate decisions. The operations can be applied to any set of treatment of intervention options. They are, therefore, generalizable to many types of settings and programs. Inherent in the system are matters of standardization and computerization that clearly enhance data processing and make possible storage and immediate retrieval. While the basic validity of the model has yet to be tested, pilot studies seem to establish reasonable reliability. Care must be taken, however, not to presume that all relevant variables necessary for quality appraisal are included.

The absence of viable mechanisms for monitoring and evaluating the quality of consultative and child care services stimulated members of the Department of Psychiatry and the Center for the Study of Health Services of Yale University and of the Connecticut Mental Health Center to work toward developing comprehensive information systems that would form the basis for a systematic approach to quality assessment in those two areas. Their work represents an extension of a collaborative relationship that began in 1969 with the Psychiatric Utilization Review and Evaluation (PURE) project. That project focused on developing a model for patient care evaluation in mental health programs, particularly as applicable to a general psychiatric population served by community mental health centers. The activities of the project involved attending to the following issues: data and data requirements for patient care evaluation (Riedel et al. 1972; Brenner and Myers 1974); methods for constructing explicit criteria for monitoring the quality of patient care (Riedel et al. 1971; Tischler and Riedel 1973; Tischler 1974); mechanisms for case review and the selection of cases for review (Goldblatt et al. 1973a; Goldblatt 1974; Brauer 1974); the use of special studies and outcome studies as integral components of a patient care evaluation system (Tischler, Henisz, and Myers 1972a; Tischler et al. 1972b; Goldblatt et al. 1973b; Astrachan et al. 1972; Schwartz, Myers, and Astrachan 1973a; Weissman et al. 1973; Schwartz, Myers, and Astrachan 1974; Henisz et al. 1974; Weissman and Paykel 1974; Schwartz and Myers 1974); and institutional issues having impact on the process of patient care evaluation (Tischler 1974; Goldblatt, Henisz, and Tischler 1974).

The activities of the PURE project, in turn, stimulated a good deal of interest within the mental health center to further refine the evaluative process. Efforts were undertaken to evaluate the efficiency of CMHC's case-selection mechanisms (Henisz et al. 1974), to develop a methodology for establishing norms for length of stay (Weiner and Levine 1975), and to test an instrument for the prospective screening of patients being considered for hospitalization (Flynn and Henisz 1975). Empirical methods for assaying the validity of normative criteria were formulated and tested (Kirstein et al. 1975; Kirstein, Weissman, and Prusoff 1975). The use of epidemiologic and ecologic analyses as adjuncts to patient care evaluation was expanded (Tischler et al. 1975).

Paralleling these activities have been efforts on the part of CMHC to modify and expand its data and information systems to enhance their utility as quality appraisal mechanisms. This has included the implementation of a problem-oriented record (Williams et al. 1973) and the development of information systems to monitor both indirect and child care services (Cytrynbaum 1974; Cytrynbaum in press). These latter two developments are particularly germane in this presentation.

An Information System for Monitoring
Consultative Services

In the area of consultative services, work has focused on:

1. developing a conceptual, rational and descriptive overview of the consultation process as a means of identifying and defining the critical parameters for inclusion in a data base;
2. creating a data and information system to record and display the minimal information required for a suitable professional review;
3. defining preliminary, operational criteria to be used as standards in the review and evaluation of case-oriented consultation activities; and,

4. proposing specific mechanisms to select consultation activities or indirect service projects for more systematic in-depth review (Cytrynbaum 1974).

An information system recording information on CMHC-sponsored, indirect-service consultation activities, and preventive programs has been developed. It includes a Project Registration Form, an Indirect Service Contract Form, and a Narrative Progress Record (Cytrynbaum 1974). This minimal but adequate system provides enumerative and descriptive information on the consultation process as a temporary social system and includes:

1. a procedure for recording base identification information on the consultee and the consultee organization;
2. a set of precoded categories for noting initial presenting problems as reported by different consultees as well as anticipated consultant intervention and consultation objectives;
3. a mechanism for recording the frequency of ongoing contacts between the consultant and consultee as well as the type of indirect service rendered; and,
4. a process for descriptively recording the effectiveness and outcome of the consultation.

Criteria for assessing the adequacy, appropriateness, and effectiveness of case-oriented consultations have been formulated by a panel of experts and transformed into a checklist for the Review of Consultation Activities (Cytrynbaum 1974).

The Children's Assessment Package (CAP)

The Children's Assessment Package provides basic data on:

1. sociodemographic variables
2. physical health and developmental history variables
3. presenting problems and behavior parameters
4. family assessment dimensions
5. school/family relationships
6. census tract and ecological data on the neighborhood and the immediate community
7. child's functioning as a student in school

The assessment of an individual child incorporates four sets of data. The MSIS Children's Admission Form completed by intake staff is utilized for recording the history of previous contacts and the child's presenting problems. Information is obtained in a checklist format on: previous contact with mental health, retardation, or related services; problems having to do with physical functions; retarded developmental progress; school functioning; school relations; child abuse; problem duration; and others.

This form is supplemented by a developmental history completed by the child's parents. Emphasis is on developmental landmarks, the emotional climate for mother, father, and child during the prenatal and postnatal periods, and on father's involvement with both mother and child during the neonatal period.

Standardized information on the child's behavior[1] and academic performance in the school setting is obtained from the teacher or an appropriate school representative. Additional information and medical history are obtained from the pediatrician or family physician or appropriate medical clinic. These two sources of data broaden the evaluation of physical and behavioral or psychological difficulties. Thus, the evaluation of the individual child includes the perspectives of a number of important figures in the child's life—clinician, parents, teacher, and physician.

Next, major attention is given to assessing family functioning and identifying recent life events that may have stressed the family system and precipitated family dysfunction. A Family Assessment Form is used to determine the nature of and basic character of family dynamics as well as of the marital, parent-child, and child-child relationships.[2] Information is obtained for an assessment by intake or clinical staff.

In addition to the evaluation of family interactional patterns, information is obtained from the family via the Significant Life Events Form regarding the possible occurrence of life crises during the year prior to seeking help. These events are presented in relation to: the family (e.g., death of an important person, serious money problems, birth of a child, family moved to another home, etc.); the mother and father (e.g., emotional, physical health, or work-related problems); and the child (e.g., child left home to live elsewhere, child had serious physical health problems, child injured by physical abuse, female child became pregnant, etc.).

Finally, the analysis of social and community factors includes a broad assessment of sociopsychological and ecological factors that may influence the functioning of the family. Included here are:

1. *Basic Background and Demographic Information.* The MSIS Children's Admission Form completed by intake staff will serve as the basis for obtaining certain demographic data including race, age, family composition, marital status, education of child, and family income. This material is supplemented by information obtained from the parents on the Family Background Form *in re*: the family's religion, the language spoken in the home, and the type of employment and level of education for both mother and father.

2. *Social Stress Indices.* Information is obtained from the Family Background Form regarding movement history (number of times the family has moved in the past five years, extent of family disruption resulting from move to new residence, etc.), the type and quality of present housing, the degree of job

satisfaction for mother and father, and the degree of satisfaction with level of education for mother and father.

3. *Social Support Network.* This position of the assessment is aimed at determining to what extent various social supports are available to the family. Several variables are utilized in evaluating the social support network such as the extent to which the family (including extended family) or supports outside the family are present in relation to child care needs and the availability of various family, friends, and/or community resources when special problems arise (i.e., concerning family, health, financial, or child-related difficulties).

4. *Family/School Relationships.* In addition to the clinician's assessment of school-related difficulties and the assessment of the child by school personnel, the Parent's Report on Family/School Relationships is included to obtain the family's view of the school program and of their child in relation to the school setting. Parents are asked to rate a series of questions that include such items as: my child likes to go to school; the difficulty my child is having is the fault of the teacher; the school authorities blame the family for my child's difficulties; my child trusts adults at school; my child is hard to control at school; no one in the school system cares what happens to my child and whether he/she learns anything; and my child needs a special class or teacher. With the inclusion of this information from the family, a comparison of school-related data provided by clinician, teacher, and the child's parents forms a broad basis for understanding the multiple dimensions of the child's school experience and the nature of the relationship between school and family.

CAP is, therefore, intended as a comprehensive psychosocial data system for children and families. It should be noted that many of the system's components can be used as measures of intermediate and long-term outcome. Thus before- and-after evaluation of service studies, as well as of comparative impact studies, across different setting or client populations, can be carried out.

In order to complete the data system, it is necessary to record direct and indirect service interventions over time. Currently, direct and indirect service contacts with children, their families, and relevant human-service agencies or facilities (such as schools) are recorded continuously using modified versions of the MSIS Direct and Indirect Service Contact Forms. These forms provide basic identification information on: the service deliverers involved; the direct or indirect service project; the consultee service recipient; the data, type, time, and manner of contact; the type of service delivered, and the service recipients present during the contact. Currently, these data are keypunched and stored on a monthly basis. Periodic reports relating client characteristics such as age, race, sex, diagnosis, etc., to types of service, length of stay, etc., are presented to the appropriate administrators and staff on a regular basis. It is now possible to retrieve data pertaining to specific questions raised by administrators, clinicians, or researchers in a reasonably short turnover time.

Conclusion

Both Professional Standards Review Organization and Utilization Review requirements strongly emphasize the evaluation of process as a practical and economical approach to quality assessment. As insistence on building mechanisms for continuously assessing quality building into service delivery systems increases, and as policy decisions concerning the structure and scope of such service systems are influenced by the outputs of this monitoring, it is incumbent upon us to ensure the existence of information systems that have the capability of providing, organizing, and displaying requisite data in ways that may simultaneously meet the needs of both service providers and program evaluators. Attention must also be paid to the reliability and validity of both the information obtained and the evaluative techniques utilized if there is to be a secure foundation on which service policy rests and service practices are constructed.

In this chapter, attention has been focused upon activities at the Connecticut Mental Health Center. These activities are aimed at developing an information system that will facilitate process evaluation in relation to the delivery of mental health services. Particular attention was given to areas of child care and consultative services. While the work is by no means finished, what *has* been done is meant to provide a sense of both the intent and range of ongoing activities and a look forward to the opportunity for further interchange.

Notes

1. The rating format and several of the items for assessing the child's behavior in school were derived from the work of Borgatta and Fanshel (1965).

2. Several items in this section were derived in a modified format from the Beavers-Timberlawn Family Evaluation Scale (Beavers, 1973). We were also influenced by personal correspondence with the Philadelphia Child Guidance Clinic.

References

Astrachan, B.M.; Adler, D.; Brauer, L.; et al. 1972. "A Checklist for the Diagnosis of Schizophrenia." *British Journal of Psychiatry* 121:529-539.

_____; Brauer, L.; Harrow, M.; et al. 1974. "Symptomatic Outcome in Schizophrenia." *Archives of General Psychiatry* 31:155-160.

Baldwin, J.A. 1971. "Aspects of the Epidemiology of Mental Illness: Studies in Record Linkage." *International Psychiatric Clinics* 7:7-12.

Beavers, W.R. 1973. "Family Variables Related to the Development of a Self." Dallas: Texas: Timberlawn Foundation Report Number 68.

Borgatta, E.F., and Fanshel, D. 1965. "Behavioral Characteristics of Children Known to Psychiatric Outpatient Clinics." New York: Child Welfare League of America, Inc.

Brauer, L.D. 1974. "Selection of Cases for Individual Review," in *Patient Care Evaluation in Mental Health Programs*, edited by D.C. Reidel, G.L. Tischler, and J.K. Myers. Cambridge, Mass.: Ballinger Publishing Co.

Brenner, N.H., and Myers, J.K. 1974. "Data and Data Systems for Patient Care Evaluation," in *Patient Care Evaluation in Mental Health Programs*, edited by D.C. Reidel, G.L. Tischler, and J.K. Myers. Cambridge, Mass.: Ballinger Publishing Co.

Brockbank, R. 1968. "Aspects of Mental Health Consultation." *Archives of General Psychiatry* 18:267-275.

Caplan, G. 1963. "Types of Mental Health Consultation." *American Journal of Orthopsychiatry* 33:470-481.

_____. 1970. *The Theory and Practice of Mental Health Consultation*. New York: Basic Books.

Crawford, J.L.; Morgan, D.W.; and Gianturco, D. 1974. *Progress in Mental Health Information Systems: Computer Applications*. Cambridge, Mass: Ballinger Publishing Co.

Cytrynbaum, S. 1974. "The Application of the Criteria-oriented Approach to the Review of Indirect Service Activities in a Community Mental Health Center," in *Patient Care Evaluation in Mental Health Programs*, edited by D.C. Reidel, G.L. Tischler, and J.K. Myers. Cambridge, Mass.: Ballinger Publishing Co.

_____. 1975. "Evaluation of Consultation Services," in *Program Evaluation from the Viewpoint of Patients, Front-line Workers and the Community*, edited by R. Coursey, G. Specter, B. Hunt, et al.

_____; Snow, D.; Phillips, E.; et al. 1975. "Program Analysis and Community Mental Health Services for Children," in *Mental Health in Children*, edited by D.V.S. Sankar. Westbury, N.Y.: PJD Publications.

Deloughery, G.W.; Gebbie, K.M.; and Neuman, B.M. 1971. "Consultation and Community Organization," in *Community Mental Health Nursing*, edited by G.W. Deloughery. Baltimore: Williams and Wilkins.

Derogatis, L.R.; Lipman, R.S.; and Cove, L. 1973. "SCL-90: An Outpatient Psychiatric Rating Scale."*Psychopharmacology Bulletin* 9:13-28.

Donabedian, A. 1966. "The Evaluation of Medical Care Programs." *Bulletin of the New York Academy of Medicine* 44:166-206.

Eiduson, B.; Brooks, S.H.; and Motto, R.L. 1966. "A Generalized Psychiatric Information Processing System." *Behavioral Science* 11:133-142.

Evenson, R.C.; Sletten, L.W.; Hedlund, J.L.; et al. 1974. "Caps: An Automated Evaluation System." *American Journal of Psychiatry* 131:531-534.

Feighner, J.P.; Robins, E.; Guze, S.B.; et al. 1972. "Diagnostic Criteria for Use in Psychiatric Research." *Archives of General Psychiatry* 26:57-63.

Flynn, H.R., and Henisz, J.E. 1975. "Criteria for Psychiatric Hospitalization:

Experience with a Checklist for Chart Review." *American Journal of Psychiatry* 132:847-850.

Fox, P.D., and Rappaport, M. 1972. "Some Approaches to Evaluating Community Mental Health Services." *Archives of General Psychiatry* 26:172-178.

Goldblatt, P.B.; Brauer, L.; Garrison, V.; et al. 1973. "A Chart Review Checklist for Utilization Review in a Community Mental Health Center." *Hospital and Community Psychiatry* 24:753-756.

_____ ; Berberian, R.M.; Goldberg, B.; et al. 1973. "Catchmenting and the Delivery of Mental Health Services." *Archives of General Psychiatry* 28:478-482.

_____ ; Henisz, J.E.; and Tischler, G.L. 1974. "Utilization Review within an Institutional Context," in *Patient Care Evaluation in Mental Health Programs*, edited by D.C. Reidel, G.L. Tischler, and J.K. Myers. Cambridge, Mass.: Ballinger Publishing Co.

_____ . 1974. "The Application of Criteria in Assessing Direct Patient Care," in *Patient Care Evaluation in Mental Health Programs*, edited by D.C. Reidel; G.L. Tischler; and J.K. Myers. Cambridge, Mass.: Ballinger Publishing Co.

Grant, R.L., and Maletzky, B.M. 1972. "Application of the Weed System to Psychiatric Records." *Psychiatry in Medicine* 3:119-129.

Grosser, C.F. 1969. "Community Development Programs Serving the Urban Poor," in *Readings in Community Organization Practice*, edited by R.M. Kramer, and H. Specht. Englewood Cliffs, N.J.: Prentice-Hall.

Hayes-Roth, F.; Longabaugh, R.; and Ryback, R. 1972. "The Problem-oriented Medical Record and Psychiatry." *British Journal of Psychiatry* 121:27-34.

Henderson, P.B.; Homann, J.; Khachaturian, Z.; et al. 1972. "Minimal Data System for Child Psychiatry." Unpublished manuscript, Pittsburgh Child Guidance Center, Pittsburgh, Pa.

Henisz, J.E.; Goldblatt, P.R.; Flynn, H.R.; et al. 1974. "A Comparison of Three Approaches to Patient Care Appraisal Based on Chart Review." *American Journal of Psychiatry* 131:1142-1144.

_____ ; Tischler, G.L.; and Myers, J.K. 1974. "Epidemiologic and Ecologic Analyses," in *Patient Care Evaluation in Mental Health Programs*, edited by D.C. Reidel, G.L. Tischler, and J.K. Myers. Cambridge, Mass.: Ballinger Publishing Co.

Hurst, W.J., and Walker, H.K. 1972. *The Problem-oriented System.* New York: Medcom Press.

Katz, M.M., and Lyerly, S.B. 1963. "Methods for Measuring Adjustment and Social Behavior in the Community: I. Rationale, Description, Discriminative Validity and Scale Development." *Psychological Report* 13:503-535.

Kessner, D.M.; Kalk, C.F.; and Singer, J. 1973. "Assessing Health Quality: The Case for Tracers." *New England Journal of Medicine* 288:189-194.

Kirstein, L.; Prusoff, B.; Weissman, M.M.; et al. 1975. "Utilization Review and Suicide Attempters: A Comparison of Explicit Criteria and Clinical Practice." *American Journal of Psychiatry* 132:22-27.

_____ ; Weissman, M.M.; and Prusoff, B. 1975. "Utilization Review and Suicide Attempters: Exploring Discrepancies between Experts' Criteria and Clinical Practice." *Journal of Nervous and Mental Disease* 160:49-56.

Laska, E.; Morril, D.; Line, S.S.; et al. 1967. "SCRIBE–A Method for Producing Automated Narrative Psychiatric Case Records." *American Journal of Psychiatry* 124:82-84.

_____ ; Simpson, G.M.; and Bank, R. 1969. "A Computerized Mental Status." *Comprehensive Psychiatry* 10:135-146.

Lee, R.L., and Jones, L.W. 1933. *The Fundamentals of Good Medical Care.* Chicago: University of Chicago Press.

Lembke, P.A. 1956. "Medical Auditing by Scientific Methods." *Journal of the American Medical Association* 162:646-655.

_____ . 1967. "Evaluation of the Medical Audit." *Journal of the American Medical Association* 199:111-118.

Lipman, R.S., et al. 1969. "Factors of Symptom Distress." *Archives of General Psychiatry* 21:328-338.

Lipp, M. 1973. "Quality Control in Psychiatry and the Problem-oriented System." *International Journal of Psychiatry* 11:355-365.

Lorr, M., and Klett, C.J. 1967. *Inpatient Multi-dimensional Psychiatric Scale.* Palo Alto, Calif.: Consulting Psychologists Press.

Mikelbank, G. 1966. "Approval by Individual Diagnosis (AID) Program, New Jersey Blue Cross." Paper presented at workshop in medical care—operation aspects, American Public Health Association, New York, November 11-12, 1966.

Miller, P.R.; Black, G.C.; Ertel, P.Y.; et al. "Psychiatric Peer Review: The Ohio System." *American Journal of Psychiatry* 131:1367-1370.

Morehead, M. 1967. "The Medical Audit as an Operational Tool." *American Journal of Public Health* 57:1643-1656.

_____ ; Donaldson, R.S.; Seravalli, M.R. 1971. "Comparisons between OEO Neighborhood Health Centers and Other Health Care Providers of Ratings of the Quality of Health Care." *American Journal of Public Health* 61:1294-1306.

Newton, P.M., and Levinson, D.T. 1973. "The Work Group within the Organization: A Socio-psychological Approach." *Psychiatry* 36:115-142.

Norman, E.C., and Forti, T.J. 1972. "A Study of the Progress and the Outcome of Mental Health Consultation." *Community Mental Health Journal* 8:261-270.

Novello, J.R. 1973. "The Problem Oriented Record in Psychiatry." *Journal of Nervous and Mental Disease* 156:349-353.

Payne, B.C. 1967. "Continued Evolution of a System of Medical Care Appraisal." *Journal of the American Medical Association* 201:536-546.

Raskin, A.; Schultenbrandt, J.; Reatig, N.; et al. 1969. "Replication of Factors of Psychotherapy in Interview, Ward Behavior and Self Report Ratings of Hospitalized Depressives." *Journal of Nervous and Mental Disease* 148:87-98.

Richardson, F.M. 1972(a). "Peer Review of Medical Care." *Medical Care* 10:29-39.

_____. 1972(b). "Methodological Development of a System of Medical Audit." *Medical Care* 10:451-462.

Richman, A., and Pinsker, H. 1972. "Utilization Review of Psychiatric Inpatient Care." *American Journal of Psychiatry* 130:900-903.

Riedel, D.C.; Tischler, G.L.; and Myers, J.K. (eds.). 1974. *Patient Care Evaluation in Mental Health Programs.* Cambridge, Mass.: Ballinger Publishing Co.

_____; Brenner, M.H.; Brauer, L.; et al. 1972. "Psychiatric Utilization Review as Patient Care Evaluation." *American Journal of Public Health* 62:1222-1228.

_____; Brauer, L.; Brenner, M.H.; et al. 1971. "Utilization Review and Evaluation in a Community Mental Health Center." *Hospital and Community Psychiatry* 22:229-232.

Roberts, L.M.; Greenfield, N.S.; and Miller, M.H. 1968. *Comprehensive Mental Health.* Madison, Wis.: University of Wisconsin Press.

Robins, E., and Guze, S.B. 1970. "Establishment of Diagnostic Validity in Psychiatric Illness." *American Journal of Psychiatry* 126:983-987.

Rogowski, A.S. 1968. "Teaching Consultation Techniques in a Community Agency," in *The Psychiatric Consultation*, edited by W. Mendell. New York: Grune & Stratton.

Rosenblum. G. 1970. "Social Intervention-Consultation to Organizations." *Mental Hygiene* 54:393-396.

Ryback, R.S., and Gardner, J.S. 1973. "Problem Formulation: The Problem Oriented Record." *American Journal of Psychiatry* 130:312-316.

Sanders, I.T. 1969. "Professional Roles in Planned Change," in *Readings in Community Organization Practice*, edited by R.M. Dramer and H. Specht. Englewood Cliffs, N.J.: Prentice-Hall, 269-277.

Schulberg, H.C., and Baker, F. 1968. "Program Evaluation Models and the Implementation of Research Findings." *American Journal of Public Health* 58:1248-1255.

_____; Sheldon, A.; and Baker, F. (eds.). 1969. *Program Evaluation in the Health Fields.* New York: Behavioral Publications.

Schwartz, C.C. 1973. "Comparing Three Measures of Mental Status: A Note on the Validity of Estimates of Psychological Disorder in Communities." *Journal of Health and Social Behavior* 14:265-273.

_____. 1974. "Psychiatric Labeling and the Rehabilitation of the Mental Patient." *Archives of General Psychiatry* 31:329-334.

_____; Myers, J.K.; and Astrachan, B.M. 1973. "The Outcome Study in Psychiatric Evaluation Research." *Archives of General Psychiatry* 29:98-102.

_____, and _____. 1974. "Outcome Studies," in *Patient Care Evaluation in Mental Health Programs*, edited by D.C. Reidel, G.L. Tischler, and J.K. Myers. Cambridge, Mass.: Ballinger Publishing Co.

Shore, M.F., and Mannino, F.V. 1969. *Mental Health and the Community: Problems, Programs and Strategies.* New York: Behavioral Publications.

Signell, K.A., and Scott, P.A. 1971. "Mental Health Consultation." *Community Mental Health Journal* 7:288-302.

Sletten, I.W.; Ernhart, C.B.; and Ulett, G.A. 1970. "The Missouri Automated Mental Status Examination: Development, Use and Reliability." *Comprehensive Psychiatry* 11:315-327.

Spitzer, R.L.; Endicott, J.; Cohen, J.; et al. 1974. "Constraints on the Validity of Computer Diagnosis." *Archives of General Psychiatry* 31:197-203.

_____, and _____. 1971. "An Integrated Group of Forms for Automated Psychiatric Case Records: A Progress Report." *Archives of General Psychiatry* 24:540-547.

Stephenson, P.S. 1973. "Judging the Effectiveness of a Consultation Program to a Community Agency." *Community Mental Health Journal* 9:253-260.

Tischler, G.L. 1974. "Developing Standards for Evaluating Direct Patient Care," in *Patient Care Evaluation in Mental Health Programs*, edited by D.C. Riedel, G.L. Tischler, and J.K. Myers. Cambridge, Mass.: Ballinger Publishing Co.

_____. 1975. "The Utilization of Mental Health Services: I. Patienthood and the Prevalence of Symptomatology in the Community. II. Mediators of Service Allocation." *Archives of General Psychiatry* 32:416-418.

_____; Henisz, J.; and Myers, J.K. 1972. "Catchmenting and the Use of Mental Health Services." *Archives of General Psychiatry* 27:389-392.

_____; Henisz, J.; Myers, J.K.; et al. 1972. "The Impact of Catchmenting." *Administration in Mental Health* 22-29.

_____, and Riedel, D.C. 1973. "A Criterion Approach to Patient Care Evaluation." *American Journal of Psychiatry* 130:913-916.

Weiner, O.D., and Levine, M. 1975. "The Process of Establishing Norms for Inpatient Units: Compiling a Report." *American Journal of Psychiatry*, in press.

Weiss, C.H. 1972. *Evaluation Research: Methods of Assessing Program Effectiveness.* Englewood Cliffs, N.J.: Prentice-Hall.

Weissman, M.M. 1975. "The Assessment of Social Adjustment." *Archives of General Psychiatry* 32:357-365.

_____; Paykel, E.S.; French, N.; et al. 1973. "Suicide Attempts in an Urban Community." *Social Psychiatry* 8:82-91.

_____, and Paykel, E.S. 1974. "Use of Special Studies: The Treatment of Suicidal Behavior," in *Patient Care Evaluation in Mental Health Programs*, edited by D.C. Riedel, G.L. Tischler, and J.K. Myers. Cambridge, Mass.: Ballinger Publishing Co.

Williams, D.H.; Jacobs, S.; Debski; et al. 1973. "Introducing the Problem Oriented Record on a Psychiatric Inpatient Unit." *Hospital and Community Psychiatry* 25:25-28.

Zusman, J., and Ross, E.R. 1969. "Evaluation of the Quality of Mental Health Services." *Archives of General Psychiatry* 20:353-357.

Zusman, J. and Slawson, M.R. 1972. "Service Quality Profile." *Archives of General Psychiatry* 27:692-698.

6

Some Problems Encountered in Attempts to Evaluate Mental Health Programs

Elaine Cumming

A useful perspective from which to begin is a slight modification of George James's (1969) classic typology of evaluation: (1) effort, (2) performance, (3) outcome, and (4) efficiency. (Although James is a perfect expositor of his own scheme, his examples, not unnaturally, always turn out to be about breast cancer and pure water supplies, or even that model of all diseases, tuberculosis; none of the problems a mental health worker faces are that simple.) The major thrust of this chapter concerns effort and performance.

Effort

Effort and performance evaluation may be grouped under the heading "good housekeeping." *Effort evaluation* is evaluation of the capacity of the service to provide care. Such an evaluation would not be too difficult if everyone who was ill were in a hospital and everyone who was out were well; in such a case, knowledge of the relevant standards for hospital care would suffice to tell us all we need to know. Since most psychiatric patients are now treated in the community, however, and since there are very few specific standards for the great variety of psychiatric treatments now in use, the task is difficult. In order to evaluate the capacity of any service to provide care, however, one must think "rates." The patience of those who know by heart how to calculate and estimate rates is solicited while this important issue is reviewed.

A *rate* is the ratio of an actual occurrence to the risk of that occurrence, calculated over a specified time, usually a year. For example, the rate of first admission among schizophrenic boys in a given catchment area is the number of 16-year-old schizophrenic boys who experience a first admission during a year, divided by all the 16-year-old boys in the catchment area. It is a simple procedure, but it is subject to two major shortcomings. First, the denominator is not always known. In other words, the number of 16-year-old boys in the catchment area might be unknown. Catchment areas whose boundaries do not match those of other jurisdictions generate this kind of problem. Wherever possible, these areas should be planned to coincide with concentrations of known populations. If the denominator problem cannot be prevented in this manner, however, there are ways of making estimates; for example, the Bureau of Census might be of help.

The second problem with rates is more insidious, and it arises through the use of inappropriate denominators. For example, for many years there was something called the "readmission rate," and it was always going up. It was calculated by dividing the number of admissions that were readmissions by all admissions. This figure was really just that: the proportion of admissions that were readmissions. The readmission rate should properly be calculated by dividing the number of readmissions by the number of people at risk of readmission (that is, by those patients who have been admitted before, have been discharged, and are now at risk of readmission). Such a rate, not too difficult to estimate, is then comparable to a first-admission rate. (It has been found, furthermore, that the readmission rate sometimes goes down while the proportion of admissions that are readmissions is going up.)

Rates of occurrences are becoming a more popular evaluation concept, but they are not exactly second nature to many mental health workers. Nevertheless, the raw material of rates is absolutely essential for evaluating how many of what kinds of people are likely or eligible to show up desiring a service. Only by knowing simple characteristics of the base population, such as age, sex, marital status, etc., is it possible to evaluate the capacity to serve. Such an evaluation is essential to good agency housekeeping—that is, knowing the job that has to be done and keeping appropriate records while doing it. Most funding bodies would probably be overjoyed to receive such information, moreover, because it is seldom routinely available.

Performance

Turning now to James's second type, performance evaluation, it can be seen that it is only a matter of slightly better housekeeping. An accounting of the actual care given by an agency is not new; annual reports are full of "output counts," but the problem with most such accountings is that they tell only what mental health workers do when they are doing their job and possibly for whom they do it. If one has an accounting of the numbers and kinds of interventions and the numbers and kinds of patients served, however, one may then ask the question "What proportion of those at risk of service actually received service?" The answer to this question reveals the rates of service utilization by various categories of people. The agency output, or care given, may look quite different when the amount of care received by those eligible to receive it is inspected (Donabedian 1969). Many questions about program and about the worrisome "redundancies and gaps" in service can be answered through such routine accountings. New forms of self-indulgence, such as excessive number of "minorities," may be found to have replaced the 33-year-old suburban housewife as the most commonly treated patient. Finally, funding agencies will probably be delighted to receive this kind of information and, in their innocence, may not know that it is just good housekeeping.

Outcome

James's next form of evaluation is research into outcome, or impact research. It is always essential for givers of service to assume that what they are doing has a favorable outcome, but it is equally essential, if this is to be more than an assumption, that properly designed research should demonstrate it. There are a number of good accounts of the range of approaches that can be used to evaluate outcome and of the problems inherent in following these approaches. Two brief comments seem in order here. First, there are times when there is absolutely no point in doing outcome studies at all. Alexander Astin pointed out long ago (1961) that when the thing to do was psychotherapy, no evidence could defer patients from demanding it and therapists from supplying it. As Astin said at that time, the issue of outcome was essentially irrelevant; psychotherapy had acquired functional autonomy and had become an end in itself. If one finds oneself in this kind of position, it might be well to save resources from something else. Suppose, for example, that sometime during the last decade it had been shown that patients treated in the mental hospital indeed did *better* than patients treated in the community, or that "consumer inputs" did *no* good and cost a lot of money. Would such messages have been heard?

The second comment on outcome evaluation is that if you are beginning to lose faith in a method of treatment, a simple before-after study may be all that is needed. There is no need for controls when the result is "no effect." (I am indebted to my colleague Peter Rossi for this insight.)

Efficiency

James's final evaluation type, the efficiency study, is really an accounting procedure which relies upon the prior existence of outcome studies. Given that desirable outcomes have been demonstrated, the efficiency study asks which is the cheapest way to achieve it. Here again, James's examples are concerned with the relative merit of fluoridating water and painting children's teeth, both of which he already knows to be valid methods of stopping dental caries. Mental health workers are seldom so happily situated, and they must often assume that the results from two different interventions are equally good, since they have no basis for choosing between them except the cost. For example, one may want to know whether to stabilize borderline schizophrenics in jobs through skill training or sociability training. First, it must be assumed that both methods work equally well. Then, the cost of the two interventions, plus the "spinoff effects" on the patient's own life, such as expected improvement in income, chances of marrying, and so on, and the spinoff effects of allocating these particular resources to the patient must be determined. The latter might include issues about whether the skill training agencies are oversubscribed or undersubscribed, whether the introduction of schizophrenics would harm the existing patient mix, and so on.

This process is easily recognizable as the so recently popular cost-benefit analysis, which according to Klarman (1965) has proved only marginally suitable for health programs because it is not possible to put dollar values on all the spinoff effects. Rossi (1972) has proposed that cost-benefit studies properly belong in the future when there are backup outcome studies on which to base it.

An encouraging new approach in the social science field is the cumulation study, which gathers all the known quantitative studies into a single statement of the probability that an effect is being observed.

Three Ubiquitous Evaluation Problems

The Goal Problem

There are some general problems encountered in evaluation processes that seem peculiarly difficult for mental health workers to solve. The first of these problems is that of defining goals. Etzione (1969), in a statement more quoted than heeded, has pointed out that goals tend to be ideals, while reality is, of course, reality.

Hence the goal of "improving the mental health of the community" is a vague and utopian, if desirable, goal. Of course, there are more realistic goals, such as reducing the length of hospitalization of schizophrenics or reducing the number of their admissions to hospitals. The problem here is, What does reducing mean? Does it mean halving it, or does it mean reducing it by 7 percent? Program administrators and evaluators are used to big goals, and one would feel silly asking for money to do something so niggardly as to reduce a rate by 7 percent. While one might not hesitate to say that the goal of a specific service is to reduce the risk of mental illness in a given population, there might be hesitancy in claiming that the program actually was reducing the incidence of schizophrenia by 3 percent. (If we were able to, however, we might get the Nobel Prize.) Because of love for the large and amorphous and embarrassment with the seeming inability to reach even modest goals, the best strategy in mental health may seem to be the stringing out of small, specific goals, or, as it is called, "management by objective." This technique, however, has its own pitfall: the endless, debilitating debate within an agency about the nature and meaning of the goals and the acceptable means toward them. One newly established mental health agency has spent literally months on such a debate, without ever seeing a patient. That particular agency's major problem was staff turnover.

The Bias Problem

There is really no good solution to the bias problem. Self-evaluations of all kinds have built-in, unavoidable conflicts of interest; because of this, the use of outside evaluators, preferably trained and if possible sophisticated, is recommended. But does this solve the problem? No doubt, the outside evaluator can come into the situation unbiased, but two facts of life soon cut in. One is that people become affiliated with one another—even trained, sophisticated people—because the most minimal interactions among people create sentiments and bonds. This means that the outside evaluator may, for reasons having to do with the logistics of the evaluation, become slightly committed (and slight commitments can create more bias than overt ones) to the points of view of some of the staff as over and against others. This is called "going native," and it should be studied more closely. There are accounts of outside evaluators "dropping out" of a research effort because they have become alienated from the program under study. But, little is known about how lesser biases are acquired by previously uncommitted evaluators and how they manifest themselves in results, reports, and recommendations.

As mental health programs are inevitably value-suffused, it could happen, for example, that an evaluator would find the core values of the program somewhat alien. This might occur in cases where the program is designed for the treatment of a problematical form of deviance, like sex offenses. In such a situation, the evaluator might feel most in sympathy with people somewhat peripheral to program policy, like accountants or personnel staff, and perhaps unwittingly absorb their biases about the program and the people who run it. Possibly replication by different evaluators is part of the answer.

Interpretation Problems

A particular pitfall for mental health workers is the interpretation of results. In many housekeeping evaluations, the problem of alternative interpretations is obvious—"Why don't the poorest people come?" for example. The solution is often equally obvious, or at least different interpretations can be kept in mind and tested. The worst problems arise when no alternative interpretations are immediately clear. Even when there are controls, effects might be artifacts or they might be properly attributable to variables that have not been measured or that cannot be separated empirically from other variables. Such ambiguities arise because many mental illnesses are of obscure etiology and the treatments themselves are, as it were, multivariate; also it cannot always be determined which aspect of the treatment achieved the result.

A good example of the doubt that can arise in interpreting even a housekeeping type of finding is evidenced in an early report from New York State by Brill and Patton (1962). They observed that among patients who had had multiple admissions to mental hospitals, those who had the shortest stays had the longest periods in the community. This finding was interpreted to mean that long stays in the hospital in some way affected the patient adversely, so that the risk of relapse was greater than it would have been if stay had been brief. An alternative explanation, however, is that onset and relapse are at least partly determined by some endogenous cyclic process. Such an hypothesis could be examined in the light of the mathematical theory known as "renewal theory." If relapse were indeed found to fit a renewal model, the possibility of this explanation being valid would be stronger. In the meantime, although Brill and Patton's own explanation of their finding is generally accepted, the possibility must be left open that it is the result of some cyclic process of the illness. Many research findings are subject to such multiple interpretations, and sometimes, as in the case of the drift hypothesis of schizophrenia, the debate rages for years.

Once the research question has been answered, the next step is to think of all the reasons why it might be wrong. (It pays to involve the local bad guys in this scenario because they will probably think of more reasons why your findings are worthless, but it is hard to bring yourself to do it.)

In conclusion, it seems worthwhile to return to a point made in the beginning of this chapter. There is nothing more fundamental to the evaluation of a service than a profile of its rates of utilization by the various categories of people entitled to its benefits. Without such information, it is not possible to be certain that a program of care, no matter how effective and efficient, is neither trivial nor unjust.

References

Astin, A. 1961. "The Functional Autonomy of Psychotherapy." *American Psychologist* 16:75-78.

Brill, H., and Patton, R. 1962. "Clinical-Statistical Analysis of Population Changes in New York State Mental Hospitals Since Introduction of Psychotropic Drugs." *American Journal of Psychiatry* 119:20-35.

Donabedian, A. 1969 "Evaluating the Quality of Medical Care," in *Program Evaluation in the Health Field*, edited by H.C. Schulberg, A. Sheldon, and F. Baker. New York: Behavioral Publications.

Etzione, A. 1969. "Two Approaches to Organizational Analysis: A Critique and Suggestion," in *Program Evaluation in the Health Field*, edited by H.C. Schulberg, A. Sheldon, and F. Baker. New York: Behavioral Publications.

James, G. 1969. "Evaluation in Public Health Practice," in *Program Evaluation in the Health Field*, edited by H.C. Schulberg, A. Sheldon, and F. Baker. New York: Behavioral Publications.

Klarman, H. 1965. *The Economics of Health*. New York: Columbia University Press.

Rossi, P. 1973. "Testing for Success and Failure in Social Action," in *Evaluating Social Programs: Theory, Practice and Politics*, edited by P. Rossi and W. Williams. New York: Seminar Press.

7

What Congress Really Wants: A Guide to Evaluating Program Effectiveness with Examples from a Canadian Context

John Cumming

"For each fiscal year for which a CMHC receives a grant under New Sections 203 (operating and continuation), 204 (consultation and education), or 205 (conversion), the center must obligate an amount equal to at least 2 percent of its previous year's operating costs for evaluating the effectiveness of its programs in serving the needs of catchment area residents, and for reviewing the quality of services it provides."[1]

This congressional statement is not, however, totally clear. First, if one assumes that the phrase "operating costs" is used here as it is elsewhere in the Mental Health Centers Act, it states that the sum to be spent is 2 percent or more of the total annual budget, which should mean that toward the end of the fiscal years of federal support, evaluation money might approach about 8 percent of the federal contribution. In business, the process by which an individual uses other people's money to augment his or her own to achieve his or her own purposes is referred to as "leverage." The second troublesome phrase is "evaluating the effectiveness of its programs." Does Congress really mean "effectiveness" in the sense that it is used technically, which would immediately mandate outcome studies of the third type described by Elaine Cumming in the preceding chapter. It would seem not; the cost of such outcome studies is of an order that would prohibit their funding from 2 percent of the average service budget. Furthermore, there are simply not enough sophisticated professionals to staff each mental health center with even a small research group. Since it must be assumed that Congress and its advisors are aware of these facts, one may read "effectiveness" in its nontechnical sense and thus make a first assumption that Congress does not expect outcome studies of treatment modalities as a routine product of CMHCs. The final assumption is that the phrase "reviewing the quality of services" means that some evaluation money can legitimately be used for expenses incurred in meeting the requirements of New Section 201(c)(2) part A, which requires that centers establish an ongoing quality assurance program (including utilization and peer review systems).

But quality assurance is surely not all that is required. In an attempt to ferret out additional issues that require focus, illustrations will be cited from a current program in Vancouver, British Columbia, with which I am associated. In this program, the basic evaluation budget is just over 2 percent of total expenditures, and a remarkable similarity exists between the concerns of the Canadian government and those of the United States' Congress (Cumming n.d.; Cumming, Coates, and Bunton in press).

Vancouver is a beautiful city of 800,000 people. British Columbia has a system of universal medical care insurance and hospital insurance. Theoretically, and very nearly in fact, all residents are free to go to the doctor or psychiatrist of their choice and receive treatment in the office or in a general hospital for a sum which will not exceed $1 per day for hospital costs. The reasons why it has been necessary to set up an extensive public service in such a situation will not be discussed here. Suffice it to state that while universal insurance solves the financial problems of institutions and therapists, it does not guarantee that those who need services are going to get them. The basis of public mental health service in this Vancouver program is the Community Care Team, a group of about twelve who serve a population area which ranges from 15,000 to 125,000. Twelve were chosen to keep team size relatively constant and to vary the population served on the basis of expected pathology. About half of each team consists of psychiatric nurses,[a] who in the main are primary therapists. The remainder of the team consists of three senior workers (one a psychiatrist), who act mainly as consultants and supervisors, an occupational therapist, and two clerical workers. The mandate of the teams is to deal with the most seriously ill and therefore usually chronic patients. They will accept a referral from any source, and they move out to find and establish contact with the patient wherever he/she is. Most of the teams have a close informal relationship with a psychiatric unit in a general hospital, often with some shared staff. A somewhat similar relationship with our provincial hospital exists. As yet, there is a lack of an adequate range of support services, including sheltered workshops and special programs for the elderly and handicapped persons. Also, there is a housing shortage for patients, although progress is being made in this area. The Community Care Team has a close relationship with training institutions and now provides field placements for all the usual helping disciplines. There are no fees, and medication is available without cost to those who need it. The provincial government provides total funding, although there is a local management group who has a considerable input into policy formation. The service is a new one with the oldest team established a little over two years ago, and growing pains still abound. Each team sees about twelve referred people a week, adding about half of those to its own patient load and referring the others to more suitable resources. A team's case load is about 250 clients. In this program, we claimed that we would provide an alternative to the large hospital; that we would serve the poor and needy; that we would be responsive; that we would coordinate our services with other agencies; that we . . . —but let us return to

---

[a]In two Canadian provinces of which British Columbia is one, a registered psychiatric nurse has a two-year training with an emphasis on the treatment of the mentally ill. Some course work overlaps with registered-nurse training, and one can be doubly qualified by spending an additional six months.

Congress and its worries since those of our provincial government rest with whether services, such as those just described, are fulfilling promises, and these promises seem to echo some of the interests of the United States' Congress.

The main source used in trying to decide what Congress wanted was the summary of the Community Mental Health Centers Amendment of 1974, prepared with extracts from the legislative history for the National Council of Community Mental Health Centers. The method was simple. Each time a criticism of center functioning was found, it was marked, sorted into categories, and assembled so that all complaints could be studied as a group. One general point is very clear. Congress is sensitive to the fact that "The Administration, since January 1973, has proposed and urged termination of the CMHC program. . . ." They know that criticisms of mental health centers, which they believe are valid in at least some cases, weaken the position that they have taken in support of CMHCs. They want the CMHCs to examine their own functioning relative to these criticisms and to assure Congress that the criticisms are groundless, or at least that the CMHCs are taking steps to rectify the errors of their ways.

To specifics: A review of the criticisms, ordered according to the lineage devoted to them, is presented, predicated on the assumption that this is perhaps some measure of the salience in the joint congressional mind.

Accessibility of Services and Attention to People's Needs

This category occupied more congressional attention than any other. Congress wants "to make services readily accessible to all residents of the community in a manner that overcomes all barriers to the receipt of services."[2] They worry about "the very special problems in securing health care faced by minority population groups whose members have limited English-speaking ability—problems which are many times intensified by different cultural heritages which make an individual's perception of health care at variance with that of the providers of health care. . . ."[3] The committee is "disturbed" [their word] by reports that poverty centers are not often utilizing the additional funds they receive, because of their poverty designation to serve the needs of the poor in their catchment areas.[4]

This concern is not surprising. Ever since Hollingshead and Redlich (1958) demonstrated that one's position in the social class order was a very good predictor of the kind of treatment that one received for a mental illness, the finding that the poor get less (and less valued) treatment has been replicated in one form or other, probably about once for every full moon. It is therefore not good enough to treat congressional worries about accessibility of services as if they were standards and to evaluate by enumerating the steps which have been taken to meet these problems. The real need is to show that plans have been effective in combating this problem. One must first describe the population and characteristics of the catchment area in specific terms that will allow for comparison of the task and how it is to be accomplished. Basic, detailed, and up-to-date census data are essential to the task of beginning an evaluation. Feldman and Windle (1971) report the existence of a study that derived from 1970 census data the population characteristics of CMHC catchment areas in the United States.[5] For those evaluators who are located in relatively stable areas, this may be a useful document. It is hoped, too, that if it is not being updated periodically, the arrangements can be made with the National Institute of Mental Health (NIMH) to do so. At any rate, an accurate population base count is essential for much evaluation work. It is a waste of effort for each CMHC to produce these figures for itself. If the data are not available federally, CMHCs should band together, perhaps on a statewide basis, to produce them.

With a catchment census as a base, one can begin to ask the question "What are we doing?" Initially, it must be determined who comes or is referred to the center and how they compare with the total population for which responsibility is assumed. When this is done for the first time, and if there are no special devices for reaching disadvantaged groups, one may confidently expect that the poor, the elderly, and the chronically ill will be underrepresented. In Vancouver, we believe that our policy of taking a referral from anyone and moving out to offer help has influenced the population mix that is served. Since the intent was to treat a population which would otherwise be hospitalized, it was necessary to compare those accepted by the teams to those who had not been referred to the teams but who had been hospitalized, on a number of variables (such as being poor, not being married, and living in isolation) usually associated with excessive rates of hospital admissions. The results indicated that the populations were similar on these sorts of variables. The hospitalized group, as expected, showed more patients who were thought to be dangerous to themselves or others, but this was the only variable examined which distinguished the two groups (Tardiff 1975).

Comparisons that failed to find differences on demographic variables were also made between patients who were referred to the team: those who, after assessment, were accepted into the patient load and those who were not accepted. The next step, which has not yet been taken, would be to determine whether patients from different backgrounds received different kinds or amounts of treatment. An example of a study of this kind is provided by Lubin et al. (1973) in Kansas City, who demonstrated that class and caste influenced assignments to inpatient or outpatient treatment and to individual or group therapies. It is the hope of the Vancouver staff to devise a study of activities, based on the sort of categories that we understand may be used in the proposed standards for CMHCs, whose development was mandated by the same legislation under discussion. These standards, it would appear, will provide a set of descriptive categories for what goes on between helper and helped that are precise and free from the ambiguities of many of our clinical terms. To have a set of categories, within which all therapists (without regard for amount of training, discipline, or experience) can categorize their helping activities, would be a most useful tool for the evaluator.

Finally, in Vancouver we have not attempted to measure outcome. We do use the POMR (problem-oriented medical record), and in one sense this seems to me to be a preparation for using Kiresuk and Sherman's (1968) Goal Attainment Scaling techniques. We hope soon to overcome the team's reluctance to use such evaluative tools.

Relationships with the State Hospital

The category of congressional worries that produced the next largest group of items dealt with the relationships between CMHCs and state hospitals, or with what happened to patients on their way either into or out of state hospitals. Congress first reaffirmed their faith that CMHC programs have "generally been a success in creating community alternatives to state inpatient facilities for mental health care." However, they cautioned that "centers vary in the extent to which they work effectively to screen admissions to state mental hospitals and facilitate the transition of former psychiatric hospital inpatients back into the community." New Section 201(6)(1) mandates that CMHCs provide "assistance to courts and other public agencies in screening residents of the catchment area being considered for referral to a state mental health facility for inpatient treatment, to determine whether they should be so referred, and to provide, where appropriate, treatment for those people through the center as an alternative to inpatient treatment in the state facility," and further to provide "follow-up care for residents of the catchment area who have been discharged from a mental health facility." Congress somewhat plaintively expressed itself as "disturbed by the failure in many instances of CMHCs and the state mental hospitals to better integrate their systems of care" and goes on "to emphasize the role of the CMHC as an alternative to hospitalization, and to make it clear to the states that CMHCs are to provide aftercare when needed."

Here again evaluation will be of the process type. The CMHCs are going to have to demonstrate that they are involved with a sizable proportion of the patients who enter state hospitals. Nor does it seem likely that Congress will accept a decrease in a related state hospital's population as evidence of the success of a CMHC. It may well be that the events are related, but the relationship will have to be demonstrated case by case. Despite the simultaneous increase in the numbers of CMHCs and the national decline in state hospital population, most evidence indicates that the two events, although contemporary, are functionally unrelated.

Relationships between CMHCs and state hospitals have traditionally been uncomfortable at best. Yet, in order to understand the dynamics of patient flow, the CMHC must have data on the patients from its area who are admitted to state hospitals. In states with highly sophisticated central data systems perhaps this sort of information might be available centrally. (Many centers will have to do what we did in Vancouver, which was to ask the state hospital to code admissions from Greater Vancouver by our service areas, and to report to us at least numerically on patient flow. We eagerly await computerization of their patient data so that we can get further demographic details of those hospitalized for comparison with the various base populations in our service areas. All we know at present is that a comparison of the five most recent months with the same months a year ago indicates that admissions from areas with established teams have decreased by about one-third, while admissions have increased slightly in areas which are not so well served.)

In Vancouver, our relationships with the provincial hospital seem to be at least moderately good. There is some shared psychiatric staff, and in those cases the psychiatrist cares for patients from the community area in which he/she works. In two service areas, there are agreements with the provincial hospital to admit patients from the area only upon the request of the community care team. This, of course, is the ultimate challenge to the community service to demonstrate its capabilities. In the end, such mandated relationships might be the beginning of a true division of labor between state hospitals and CMHCs.

Let us pass on, however, to other categories. Fortunately, the intensity of the complaints and their focus both seem to diminish from this point.

Administrative Efficiency, Cost Control, and National Health Insurance

This category seems to have several aspects. The first of these is epitomized by Congress characterizing its present legislation as an attempt "to respond to the administration's legitimate concerns over administrative efficiency in centers and the need for centers to grow toward self-sufficiency." Indeed, congressional comment seems to support this as a central function when discussing "the need to establish national standards for centers . . . to require . . . more comprehensive services, improved management and financial administration. . . ." Let us leave administrative efficiency to the auditors, however, since this seems clearly to be part of the monitoring function of federal bureaucracy mandated by the legislation we are considering.

There is still an aspect of the comment in this area which is deeply disturbing, however. Congress speaks of the necessity "to build a system for provision of mental health services available in each community which has proper cost and quality control mechanisms prior to the enactment of national health insurance which finances mental health services."[6]

It appears that national health insurance is anticipated as a portent of the millennium when at least Congress will be able to lay down its burden of supporting this controversial cause and leave the CMHCs to provide mental health care to a population who can afford it through national health insurance. Ironically, this shift of fiscal responsibility may well deny service to just those groups which Congress is currently demanding that we demonstrate that we are serving.

In the most efficient of national insurance systems, there will always be a small minority who, usually through their own incompetence, have never been covered, or whose coverage for one or another causes has lapsed. In British Columbia, it is probable that the group who lacks medical care coverage for physician services does not exceed 3 or 4 percent of the population. Given a week or two, almost all these people could obtain entitlement for service. Yet there are times when it seems that literally all in this group are mentally ill, and when they need service, it cannot be postponed until they obtain coverage. This, of course, is not the end of the picture; fiscal control mechanisms, the schedule of procedures for which psychiatrists can charge, and many other factors combine to make insurance a bonanza for both the middle class and the treatment institution which needs a stable funding base, but a disaster for the poor. Ironically, hospitalization insurance is dependent only on residence in British Columbia for at least three months. The procedure is automatic, and thus most of the poor are effectively covered. However, you need a doctor to admit you to a hospital and who will care for you while you are there, and the poor have trouble finding one.

Consultation and Education; Relationships with Community Agencies

Consultation and education services have a new status under the new 1974 legislation. While these services have always been recommended for CMHCs, from 1974 onward they will receive ongoing federal support, even after funds are no longer available for other services. Since the phrase "consultation and education" has been used to describe a wide variety of programs, an attempt was made to find the congressional interpretation. The House of Representatives says: "Through more effective consultation and education, the center will receive more appropriate referrals, enable other caregivers to manage their clients more effectively, and enhance continuity of care, as well as extending service to underserved groups in the catchment area."[7] Again, as we have quoted before, they list as the first goal of education "to increase the visibility, identifiability and accessibility of the CMHC" and put in second place the more usually cited function "to promote mental health and to prevent emotional disturbance through the distribution and dissemination of relevant mental health knowledge."

Thus, it seems that these services are seen more as a way of realizing the basic goals of the CMHC than as primary objectives in their own right. If this is the case, evaluation of these services becomes somewhat simpler. In Vancouver, we did a very primitive study which simply sought to determine the degree of satisfaction with our services held by agencies who had referred patients to us. Not unexpectedly, they complained of a lack of feedback on the patient's progress. This seems to be a universal failing. We are gratified, however, that they rated us high on responsiveness, saying that in times of crisis the team's reaction was prompt and sufficient. Other studies which should be done have not yet been carried out. These include how agency referrals compare with the characteristics of our catchment area population and how they differ from people who seek help on their own. Also needed is more information about the numbers and kinds of mental health problems which agencies are prepared to accept, so that a service map of the area may be developed. While procedures in Vancouver are set up to ensure that referrals at least arrive at the agency to which they are referred, as yet no studies have been made of the outcome of these referrals from the point of view of either client or agency satisfaction. The importance of continuity of care is a consideration which has been raised several times by Congress. Ways need to be devised to study the characteristics of those who slip through the treatment net and to evaluate the circumstances that seem to be associated with these losses.

Miscellaneous

My list of categories—and perhaps the reader—is now exhausted. All that remains are a few unrelated items. I note that the Act mandates reports to the Department of Health, Education and Welfare (HEW) and to the public within the catchment area. From the list of items to be covered, it seems that many of the studies mentioned above would be very useful in compiling these reports. Or, looked at in another way, a moderate expansion of the data collection necessary for this report would enable one to make analyses which would answer some of the questions proposed here.

One final point: the 1974 Act mandates that HEW develop and provide standards for CMHCs. This task is in process, and it is hazardous to comment on it, especially since others have later information than I have. Yet, it was most encouraging to see, at least in preliminary work, that an attempt is being made to have CMHCs describe their activities in terms which are simple and precise. The question would not be "Do you have a children's program?" but rather "What activities do you engage in during the treatment of children?" Further, the description would be structured into terms that would cut through the usual language that we use to help us not to think about what we are doing. I even have some hope that we might permanently get rid of my least-liked term, "prevention." Since almost nothing is known about the prevention of mental illness, the term is commonly used to describe a program which we want to carry out but which we fear would not be acceptable under a more honest description. Perhaps, if one were forced into a more accurate and down-to-earth description of what she or he proposed to do and what she or he hoped to accomplish, one could even hope to evaluate it.

I am grateful to those who asked me to accept this task. It has sharpened my awareness that what is being demanded of community services in the United States is little different from that which is required in Canada, and I suspect in other countries where psychiatry is leaving its traditional public hospital base.

Notes

1. New Section 206(c)(4). Community Mental Health Centers Amendment of 1975, Title III of PL 94-63.
2. Senate Bill 93-1137, p. 47.
3. Senate Bill 93-1137, p. 6.
4. Senate Bill 93-1137, pp. 8-49; and H 93-1524, p. 74.
5. The document referred to by Feldman and Windle is DHEW Publication Number (HSM) 75-9051 (1971).
6. House Bill 93-1161, p. 31.
7. House Bill 93-1524, p. 74.

References

Cumming, J. "The Vancouver Plan." Mimeo. n.d. Available from Community Care Services Society, 1019 Wharf Street, Victoria, British Columbia.

_____ , Coates, D., and Bunton, P. "Community Services in Vancouver: The Initial Phase of Planning and Implementation." *Canadian Psychiatric Association Journal.* In press.

Hollingshead, A.B., and Redlich, F.C. 1958. *Social Class and Mental Illness.* New York: John Wiley & Sons, Inc.

Kiresuk, T.J., and Sherman, R.E. 1968. "Goal Attainment Scaling: A General Method for Evaluating Community Mental Health Programs." *Community Mental Health Journal* 4: 443-453.

Lubin, B., Hornstra, R.K., Lewis, R.V., and Vechtel, B.S. 1973. "Correlates of Initial Treatment Assignment in a Community Mental Health Center." *Archives of General Psychiatry* 29: 497-500.

Tardiff, K. 1975. "Comparison of Social and Psychopathological Characteristics of Patients Referred to Community Care Teams and to Hospitals." Greater Vancouver Mental Health Service: Research report no. 7 (March).

8 Evaluation of Patient Outcome: An Overview of Approaches

Elizabeth W. Markson

Evaluation of the impact of treatment programs, specifically in terms of patient outcome, has not suffered from inattention but rather from complexity and diversity of aims, from differences in criteria, from variations in solution, and, occasionally, from cavalier resolution. This chapter presents a brief overview of various "off the shelf" approaches to patient outcome used in the past two decades. This survey is not all-inclusive but rather highlights basic dimensions of patient outcome considered in a variety of studies.[1]

Because the scope of patient outcome evaluation is so vast, an outline of some current approaches seems useful. These include the following.

1. Client comments on benefits received from a particular program—a more stringent version of this is client evaluations of benefits received using standardized interviews or scales.

2. Client self-ratings on psychopathology.

3. "Accountability audits," including biometric reports such as data on patient movements into or out of treatment.

4. Social experiments, characterized by random assignment of clients to alternative treatments or to control and experimental groups (or patchwork variations thereof necessitated by circumstance), and standardized measures of "success" or "failure."

5. Survey of released patients, or their families, or general population groups for the purpose of ascertaining the effect of a mental health program on specific persons or on part of or all of a community or catchment area, again usually employing standardized measures.

6. Case studies—in which detailed descriptions are prepared for one or more cases and reviewed for meaningful clusters of information that may be generalized to other people or groups.

7. Clinical evaluations, using professional judgments or a scale, of changes in the patient, of ward rating scales of patient behavior, of social workers' ratings, etc.

8. Cost-analytic techniques, including cost-benefit analyses encompassing evaluation of the relative effectiveness of various approaches in terms of attainment of a specific goal—this is often expressed in dollars on both sides of the equation (e.g., cost of the program versus economic self sufficiency of the client).

9. Cost-outcome analysis, in which client or program goals are related to criteria less tangible than money, such as release to the community.

The above listing of approaches to patient outcome, drawn from Davis (1971), highlights the point that most such models in the field of mental health assume (either explicitly or implicitly) that some aspect of the client's behavior is to be changed. Suchman (1966) has observed that the primary goal in evaluation is to determine the extent to which an activity is associated with occurrence of results. The secondary goal is to test the validity of the conclusion that the specific activity produced that effect. He further suggests that there are certain general considerations involved in the formulation of the objectives of the program that must be reflected upon prior to actual evaluation, including:

1. What are we trying to change?
2. Who is the target population?
3. What is the desired change?
4. Does the program have one objective or several?
5. What is the desired magnitude of the change?

Yet, as the above list suggests, methods of evaluations of outcome in mental health have differed considerably. Foci have encompassed psychiatric evaluations or simple clinical ratings of symptomatology (mild, moderate, severe), such as those used by Wilder et al. (1968), demographic studies of hospital use and hospital-community flow such as those by Kramer (1969, 1973), as well as purely social and anthropological analyses where, as in the early studies of Freeman and Simmons (1963), "psychiatric status and what may be described as 'medical variables' were given no place in . . . consideration of post-hospital experience of mental patients."[2] Newer techniques, such as goal attainment scaling (described in Chapter 11) and outpatient value analysis (Halpern and Binner 1972), have developed specifically in response to outcome evaluation needs. Many studies of patient outcome, however, have not followed an evaluation framework—one that studies the relationship between a specific program and the attainment of some predetermined objective or set of objectives. Very often attention has instead been placed either on one aspect or another of the patient's mental status or social functioning without reference to a specific treatment program, or conversely, on only the treatment program itself. Only infrequently has light been shed on the ways in which patient outcome and specific aspects of the program may interact. This is at least in part due to methodological difficulties inherent in such a close-grained analysis of variables.

Nonetheless, a common denominator of the majority of studies touching upon patient or ex-patient outcome remains that of behavior, although the way in which behavior has been defined varies considerably. Certainly behavioral modifications, however defined, is a goal in the treatment of the mentally ill, the alcoholic, the addicted, the retarded, and the developmentally disabled; the desired changes in these disparate groups are improved levels of functioning. It is with a selection of somewhat traditional approaches to levels of functioning of the mentally ill that this article is concerned.

Improved level of functioning as a goal of treatment is probably not one objective but several, encompassing relief of psychic distress and symptomatology when possible, enhanced physical functioning where appropriate (especially among groups with physical disabilities or problems), and improved social and economic functioning, whether within a sheltered or a community setting. Economic independence, "normal" role relationships with others in the community, and community acceptance of the patient or ex-patient would also be desired changes. In short, the aim of most mental health programs is to enhance the social and personal functioning of patients—that is, the characteristic ways in which they react to life situations (ways that are valued by the society as a whole).

Social functioning may be usefully viewed in several dimensions, including: (1) social participation, or the degree to which patients participate in a variety of activities, including voluntary associations, social activities with friends, social activities with relatives, participation in religious activities, and close friendships and love relationships; (2) work performance or employment status; and (3) perceived normality or stress producing patient behavior, as reported by the immediate family or persons in closest contact with the patient.

Personal functioning encompasses the patient's psychological well being and/or degree of pathology or mental health. A complex problem exists, in view of the fact that there is no precise definition of mental health. A wide variety of techniques has been utilized to assess its various dimensions. These range from simple face-validity measures of happiness (Bradburn and Caplovits 1965) to detailed clinical evaluations (Endicott and Spitzer 1976).

During the past two decades, a plethora of studies focusing on the fate of the released mental patient have been published, many of which have used similar, sometimes identical, measures of social adjustment after release from hospitalization and treatment. (See, for example, Freeman and Simmons 1963; Scarpetti and Dinitz 1967; Myers, Bean, and Pepper 1968; Brown et al. 1966; Dinitz, Angrist, Lefton, and Pasamanick 1962; Molholm and Dinitz 1972; Maisel 1967; Morrow and Robins 1964; Mandelbrote and Folkard 1961; Gove and Lubach 1969; Waters and Northover 1968; Pollack et al. 1968; Fakhruddin et al. 1972; Davis et al. 1972; Gove and Fain 1973; Stimpert et al. 1965). Methods of data collection have also been similar; generally, patients and/or members of the patients' families were interviewed in the community, most often by trained interviewers who were not primarily clinicians. Results on specific groups were analyzed to provide information on what sort of adaptation former patients made to the community and what the correlates of their success or failure to adjust might be. While many of these studies are indeed "old," the techniques used therein address salient variables indicative of community adjustment. Areas of particular interest for assessment of the efficacy of deinstitutionalization and community-based treatment are reviewed below.

Work Performance

Perhaps the role most consistently expected of adults (except for the elderly) in American society is work or, in sociological terms, instrumental performance. While the "normal" female work role remains more ambiguous than that of the male (and both are currently undergoing reexamination and redefinition), traditionally most authors of outcome studies have assumed that an active role in taking care of the home (and children when present) in lieu of outside employment is expected of non-gainfully employed adult women. The man or woman who, like the lilies of the field toils not, is usually not only socially visible but runs the risk of being labeled a loafer, a bum, a deviant, or at best, a "poor thing." Various measures of work performance have been devised, but most often they employ a continuum, such as that shown below, for males and for females who are not primarily wives and mothers.

Gradations of Duration and Stability of Employment Since Release

Best /   /   /   /   /   /   /   / Worst

(Worked) full time since end of treatment)   (Not gainfully employed since release)

Added to this simple multipoint scale may be means of support if unemployed or if supplemental benefits are received—the latter provides a rough indicator of the degree to which clients are "public charges." This is a question of more than passing interest to our protestant work ethic society, especially during a period of rising taxes, recession, and inflation.

Assessment of the work performance of homemakers is more difficult, but numerous attempts have been made to quantify the "usual" tasks performed by the "competent" homemaker. These include such chores as: (1) dusting, sweeping, other usual cleaning; (2) laundry, mending; (3) meal preparation; (4) grocery shopping; (5) handling household budget and monies; (6) dressing and bathing children; (7) getting children to school on time; and (8) routine discipline of children. Depending on the complexity of information desired and the population being assessed, these two basic areas—household activity and employment status—may be expanded or contracted and appropriate sets of tasks added or subtracted to fit the socioeconomic characteristics and value patterns of each group under study. (For example, a series of usual household duties developed for use with residents of East Harlem might differ in content from those developed for interviews either with residents of Chicago's Gold Coast or Cambridge's intelligentsia, where not only specific tasks but sex role expectations differ among the groups.)

Social Participation

In contrast with work and household task performance, it is obvious that there are many more subcultural variations in normative definitions of appropriate conduct with respect to social participation in the community (Myers and Bean 1968). Put differently, social participation is affected by social class, ethnicity, marital status, length of time in community or neighborhood, urban versus rural residence, religious ties, personal preference, and a host of other factors *aside from* psychopathology. With different degrees of caution, the following types of indicators of social participation have been used in impact studies: (1) regular participation in voluntary association, such as club, union, lodge, professional society, or special interest group; (2) social activities with at least one friend within a specified time period; (3) attendance at religious services within a specified time period; (4) knowledge of at least one neighbor to say hello to and to exchange house visits with; and (5) possession of at least one hobby or spare time activity that is engaged in at least once within a specified time period.

Caution should be used in establishing a set of social participation items or interpreting a certain level of activity as *ipso facto* normal. One instrument, for example, the Community Adaptation Schedule (CAS) (Roen and Burnes 1968), includes a series of items on social participation and has established norms against which the performance of mentally ill or ex-patients may be compared. The CAS, while unusual in that norms for the nonmentally ill have been developed for comparison, used as its reference point of normal behavior the responses of middle-class mental health professionals—responses likely to differ from those of primarily lower-class patients receiving treatment in a mental hospital.

Burden on Community, Perceived Normality of
Behavior, or Apparent Psychopathology

This unwieldy heading reflects variations in terminology for a means of assessing the way in which patient behavior is interpreted by patients' family members or others in close contact. One of the most widely used techniques to assess perception was developed by Katz and his associates at the National Institute of Mental Health (NIMH) (Katz and Lyerly 1963; Lorr 1966) during the 1960s. It encompasses both patients' symptomatology and social behavior. Self-ratings and ratings by mental health professionals, semiprofessionals, and relatives of mentally ill patients may be made using this or similar sets of scales (See for example, Stewart et al. 1969; Michaux et al. 1969; Levine et al. 1970; Simmons and Freeman 1963; Dinitz et al. 1963.) A very similar technique, the Community Adjustment Scale, has been devised by Ellsworth et al. (1968) and like the Katz scales, encompasses both the social and symptom areas of behavior. Another popular rating scale, the MACC, also developed by Ellsworth (1971), permits a behavioral rating in layperson's terms on such aspects of conduct as "is he sullen?" and "does she spend her time alone?" This scale may be easily completed by family members, ward attendants, or others without clinical training but familiar with the patient.

The extent to which patients' behavior represents a "burden" on their families or the community has also been assessed and is perhaps of more interest as community-based treatment becomes the norm rather than the exception for the mentally ill and the retarded. The amount of distress experienced by the family as a result of the patient's presence or return home encompasses management problems in dealing with the patient, amount of time missed from work as a result of the patient's needs/demands, familial physical and psychic disorders, and economic support problems (Brown et al. 1966; Hamilton 1968; Grad and Sainsbury 1968). While indicators such as these are extremely valuable in showing how specific people (or group of people) are *perceived* by those around them, the extent to which family members or others in close contact with the patient are reliable reporters of the patient's actual condition or level of functioning remains open to question. Reports by Laing and Esterson (1964), Markson (1972), and Miller (1971) indicate a "Rashomon" effect at work; differences in perception between the patient and the family or the patient and the caretaker are notable. For example, families are more likely to blame the patients themselves for their illness, while patients cite familial or environmental stresses (Miller 1971). Even simple reports of ability for self-care are subject to variation; ward level staff may consistently view patients as less physically competent than do patients or their relatives (Markson 1972). Whether, indeed, the patients or those around them are more veracious is moot. Parenthetically, what seems clear is that the *congruency* of patient versus other reports on behavior is crucially related to outcome; when all *agree* that the patient does or does not need treatment, successful community adjustment is most likely to occur (Miller 1967).

Personal Integration

There is, of course, no neat dividing line between social functioning and psychological functioning—the two are inextricably confounded. An excellent illustration of the close relationship between these two dimensions is provided by an examination of normality of behavior as perceived by one's family. Items like those included in the scales developed by Katz et al. (1963), Ellsworth et al. (1968), Simmons and Freeman (1963), etc. indicate the extent to which the patient fails at a number of "normal" role responsibilities and show, either tacitly or explicitly, how much of a burden they may be to their families as well as how much they demonstrate overtly psychotic behavior. The approaches to patient outcome reviewed below are closely related to social functioning but focus primarily upon the psychic state of the respondent. Since methods of designating psychological states vary considerably—both in assumptions and levels of complexity—they are arbitrarily divided into two sections here: (1) global self-assessment of morale and happiness, and (2) delineations of mental status based upon models of psychopathology.

Global Measures of Happiness

Happiness, like health, is highly valued in American society and is implicitly or explicitly a salient variable in assessment of morale. At its grossest level, happiness is a measure of psychological well-being or "mental health." Yet, while one may speak of being more or less happy (essentially a continuum), at present there is no agreement about what the core definition of happiness (or, for that matter, morale or mental health) is. Despite the lack of a firm reference point for the true meaning of happiness—if, indeed, it is an absolute—there is some suggestion (Bradburn and Caplovitz 1965) that self-assessments of good spirits have face validity, are easy to obtain, and reflect individual overall role adjustment.

Bradburn and Caplovitz (1963, 1965) have indicated that positive and negative feelings, each correlating positively to respondents' self reports of happiness, are independent of one another rather than following from a consubstantial base. Put differently, the fact that positive and negative feelings represent separate dimensions suggests a modification of the Bentham notion of "happiness is the absence of pain" to a formulation more like that of J.S. Mill where "the experience of negative feelings is offset by the experience of several positive feelings" (Bradburn 1963).

Thus it would appear that such symptoms as anxiety—usually indicative of at least mild mental disorder—*add* to negative feelings but do *not* subtract from positive feelings. Simply put, if one reports feeling unhappy and also reports a number of negative feelings, one is likely to be anxious. Yet anxiety is not basic to unhappiness; what is significant is the affect balance (or ratio of positive to negative feelings). With enough positive feelings, one may be anxious and happy. A simple technique for assessing "well-being,"—self reports of happiness—has been used to assess "normals" (Gurin et al. 1960; Bradburn and Caplovitz 1965), schizophrenics (Alexander 1967), and psychiatrically impaired elderly people (Markson 1975). These self reports are an integral aspect of many measures of morale.

Clinical Ratings of Psychopathology

A vast number of techniques have been developed through which psychopathology may be assessed. These differ in complexity and detail—ranging from the Global Adaptation Scale (GAS) developed by Spitzer et al. and described briefly in Chapter 10 and the Brief Psychiatric Rating Scale (Gorham and Overall 1962) (BPRS)—a twenty-six item inventory completed by a clinician after interviewing a patient, to the Psychiatric Evaluation Form (Endicott and Spitzer 1976). Because the number of rating methods by which psychopathology may be assessed is so large, it is impractical to review them here. [Two useful sources for rating scales of patient symptomatology and clinical outcome are Lyerly (1973) and *Mental Measurements Yearbook*, which reviews many objective scales and is updated periodically (Buros 1972).] Patient self-ratings on psychopathology also provide a means of assessing outcome, but they generally require either psychologically naive or treatment-motivated respondents if answers are to be other than normative. Many long-term, or treatment-wise, people may be less than candid if they are aware of the possible consequences—including rehospitalization—of giving "sick" responses. Choice of technique and interpretation of results are complex; responses that may be associated with mental disorder in one group may be the norm for the other, never ill, groups (Dohrenwend 1976).

What Techniques?

With a wide variety of "off-the-shelf" approaches that have been used to assess patient outcome, which are most appropriate to use? Obviously, in part, the choice of outcome measures is contingent on the interests of the investigator, the amount of money available for assessment of outcome (interviews are expensive as are lengthy ratings by clinically trained professionals), as well as the general validity of the techniques implied by the approach. In evaluation of patient outcome, the criteria for evaluation of a program, suggested by Suchman at the beginning of this chapter are especially relevant. Assuming that the goal of a specific mental health program is to change behavior, it seems crucial to determine a priori what the desired change in behavior may be. This paper has reviewed several aspects of behavior that reflect one aspect or another of functioning, including social participation, work, perceived normality of behavior, and clinical assessments. Depending on the objectives of the particular program being evaluated, one or another aspect of functioning may be the "best" indicator of its impact upon patients. That the choice of outcome indicators be realistically related to the program and its specific clientele is also important—what kind and how much change can be settled for, as indicators of favorable outcome for patients, are basic questions in any program evaluation. Relatively simple techniques, such as those outlined here, are not only inexpensive, but permit before-after comparisons of people as they move through mental health programs.

Notes

1. For an overview of social adjustment measures, see Weissman (1975).
2. Freeman and Simmons (1963), p. 4.

References

Alexander, W. 1967. "Some Sociological Aspects of Psychological Well-being in a Schizophrenic Population." Doctoral dissertation, Syracuse University.

Bradburn, N. 1963. "In Pursuit of Happiness." Chicago: NORC Report 92.

_____ , and Caplovitz, D. 1965. *Reports on Happiness.* Chicago: Aldine Press.

Brown, G.W., et al. 1966. *Schizophrenics and Social Care: A Comparative Follow-up Study of 339 Schizophrenic Patients.* London: Oxford Press.

Buros, O.K., ed. 1972. *Seventh Mental Measurements Yearbook.* New York: Gryphon Press.

Davis, A.E., et al. 1972. "The Prevention of Hospitalization in Schizophrenia: Five Years after an Experimental Program." *American Journal of Orthopsychiatry* 42:375-388.

Davis, H.R. 1971. "The Use of Program Evaluation in Front Line Services." Washington, D.C.: U.S. Government Printing Office, DHEW Publication No. (HSM) 71-9057.

Dohrenwend, B.P. 1976. "Sociocultural and Socio-psychological Factors in the Genesis of Mental Disorders." *Journal of Health and Social Behavior* 16:365-392.

Ellsworth, R.; Foster, L.; Childers, B.; and Krocker, D. 1968. "Hospital and Community Adjustment as Perceived by Psychiatric Patients, Their Families and Staff." *Journal of Consulting and Clinical Psychology*, monograph supplement, 32: 1- 41.

Ellsworth, R.B. 1971. *The MACC Behavioral Adjustment Scale: Revised 1971.* Los Angeles: Western Psychological Services.

Endicott, J., and Spitzer, R. 1976. "Clinical Evaluation and Patient Outcome," in *Trends in Mental Health Evaluation*, edited by E. Markson and D. Allen. Lexington, Mass.: D.C. Heath.

Fakhrudden, A.K.M. et al. 1972. "A Five Year Outcome of Discharged Chronic Psychiatric Patients." *Canadian Psychiatric Association Journal* 17:433-435.

Freeman, H.E., and Simmons, O.G. 1963. *The Mental Patient Comes Home.* New York: John Wiley & Sons, Inc.

Gorham, D.R., and Overall, J.E. 1962. "The Brief Psychiatric Rating Scale." *Psychological Reports* 16:799-812.

Gove, W., and Lubach, J. 1969. "An Intensive Test Program for Psychiatric Inpatients: A Description and Evaluation." *Journal of Health and Social Behavior* 10:225-236.

Gove, W.R., and Fain, R. 1973. "The Stigma of Mental Health Hospitalization: An Attempt to Evaluate Its Consequences." *Archives of General Psychiatry* 28:494-500.

Grad, J., and Sainsbury, P. 1968. "The Effects that Patients Have on Their Families in a Community Care and a Control Psychiatric Service: A Two Year Follow-up." *British Journal of Psychiatry* 114:265-278.

Gurin, G.; Verof, J.; and Feld, S. 1960. *Americans View Their Mental Health.* New York: Basic Books.

Halpern, J., and Binner, P.R. 1972. "A Model for an Output Value Analysis of Mental Health Programs." *Administration in Mental Health* 40-51.

Hamilton, M.W. 1968. "The Hospital and the Household," in *Community Mental Health: An International Perspective*, edited by R.H. Williams and L.D. Ozarin. San Francisco: Jossey-Bass.

Katz, M.M., and Lyerly, S. 1963. "Methods for Measuring Adjustment and Social Behavior in the Community: I. Rationale, Description, Discrimination Validity and Scale Development." *Psychological Reports* 13:503-535.

Kiresuk, T. 1976. "Goal Attainment Scaling at a Community Mental Health Service," in *Trends in Mental Health Evaluation*, edited by E. Markson and D. Allen. Lexington, Mass.: D.C. Heath.

Kramer, M. 1969. *Application of Mental Health Statistics: Uses in Mental Health Programmes of Statistics Derived from Psychiatric Services and Selected Vital and Morbidity Records.* Geneva, Switzerland: World Health Organization.

_____ ; Taube, C.A.; and Redick, R.W. 1973. "Patterns of Use of Psychiatric Facilities by the Aged: Past, Present and Future," in *Psychology of Adult Development and Aging*, edited by C. Eisdorfer and M.P. Lawton. Washington, D.C.: American Psychological Association.

Laing, R., and Esterson, A. 1964. *Sanity, Madness and the Family.* London: Tavistock.

Levine, H.I., et al. 1970. "The Aftercare of Schizophrenics: An Evaluation of Group and Individual Approaches." *Psychiatric Quarterly* 44:296-304.

Lorr, M. 1966. *Explorations in Typing Psychotics.* New York: Pergamon Press, Inc.

Lyerly, S.B. 1973. *Handbook of Psychiatric Rating Scales*, 2d ed. Bethesda, Md.: NIMH.

Maisel, R. 1967. "The Ex-mental Patient and Rehospitalization: Some Research Findings." *Social Problems* 15:18-24.

Mandelbrote, B.M., and Folkard, S. 1961. "Some Factors Related to Outcome and Social Adjustment in Schizophrenia." *Acta Psychiatrica Scandinavica* 37:223-235.

Markson, E. 1972. "Growing Old in America: Some Structural Problems: Current Comment: Symposium on the Aging Poor." *Syracuse Law Review* 23:60-68.

Michaux, W.W., et al. 1969. *The First Year Out: Mental Patients after Hospitalization.* Baltimore: Johns Hopkins Press.

Miller, D. 1967. "Retrospective Analysis of Posthospital Mental Patients' Worlds." *Journal of Health and Social Behavior* 8:136-140.

_____. 1971. "Worlds that Fail," in *Total Institutions*, edited by S.E. Wallace. New Brunswick, N.J.: Trans-action Books.

Molholm, L.H., and Dinitz, S. 1972. "Female Patients and Their Normal Controls." *Archives of General Psychiatry* 27:606-610.

Morrow, W.R., and Robins, A.J. 1964. "Family Relations and Social Recovery of Psychotic Mothers." *Journal of Health and Human Behavior* 5:14-24.

Myers, J.K., and Bean, L. (with M. Pepper) 1968. *A Decade Later: A Follow-up of Social Class and Mental Illness.* New York: John Wiley & Sons, Inc.

Pasmanick, B.; Scarpitti, F.R.; and Dinitz, S. 1967. *Schizophrenics in the Community.* New York: Appleton-Century-Crofts.

Pollack, M.; Levenstein, S.; and Klein, D.F. 1968. "A Three Year Post Hospital Follow-up of Adolescent and Adult Schizophrenics." *American Journal of Orthopsychiatry* 38:94-109.

Roen, S.R., and Burnes, A.J. 1968. *CAS: Community Adaptation Schedule: Preliminary Manual.* New York: Behavioral Publications.

Stewart, A., et al. 1969. "Patterns of Adjustment of Discharged Patients as Measured by Mailed Questionnaires." *Community Mental Health Journal* 5:314-319.

Stimpert, W.E., et al. 1966. "A Description of Psychiatric Patients Five Years after Treatment." *Social Work* 11:78-86.

Suchman, E. 1966. "A Model for Research and Evaluation on Rehabilitation," in *Sociology and Rehabilitation*, edited by B. Sussman. Washington, D.C.: American Sociological Association, pp. 52-70.

Waters, M.A., and Northover, J. 1968. "Rehabilitated Long-stay Schizophrenics in the Community." *British Journal of Psychiatry* 111:258-267.

Weissman, M. 1975. "The Assessment of Social Adjustment." *Archives of General Psychiatry* 32:357-365.

Wilder, J.; Kessel, M.; and Cowlfield, S. 1968. "Follow-up of a 'High Expectations' Halfway House." *American Journal of Psychiatry* 124:103-109.

Clinical Evaluation of Patient Outcome

Jean Endicott and *Robert L. Spitzer*

In earlier chapters the term "evaluation" has been used very broadly. In this chapter, evaluation procedures which are useful in helping to determine the relative efficacy of two or more treatment approaches will be discussed.

An investigator wishing to compare different treatment approaches, with an aim toward improving the delivery of mental health services, must determine both the design of the study and the measures to be used as criterion indices of improvement. Unless careful attention is paid to selecting the appropriate design and measures, the value of the results will be extremely limited and even potentially misleading.

Problems of Design

There are three critical issues to be considered in determining the appropriate design for an evaluation study. First, should the design be naturalistic or experimental? Second, should all subjects be involved, or should there be specially selected samples of subjects? And finally, should the evaluations be routine therapists' evaluations or special evaluations by therapists or independent assessors?

Naturalistic versus Experimental Design

The first issue to be faced is whether a naturalistic or experimental design is to be employed. In a naturalistic design, all aspects of patient selection and treatment assignment are left to the vagaries of usual clinical practice. The naturalistic design has great appeal for administrators: None of their usual operations need to be disturbed. Therapists are not told whom they can treat, for how long, in what way, etc. Patients do not need to be told that they are being selected or assigned to treatments on the basis of a research protocol, and they are not required to give informed consent for the treatment selected.

In contrast, in an experimental design both the criteria for selecting subjects and treatment assignment are carefully controlled and clearly specified. Of necessity, an experimental research protocol always requires changing usual clinical procedures. Instead of assigning a patient to a treatment that the clinician is convinced is optimal for that patient, a protocol must be followed which implies that the optimal treatment is unknown and which may result in a patient being assigned to a treatment that the clinician feels is clearly inappropriate. For example, in a study of day versus inpatient hospitalization (Herz et al. 1971), the protocol required a random assignment of all study patients to either day or inpatient care within the first few days of hospitalization. Although clearly suicidal and violent patients had been excluded, many therapists felt uncomfortable placing patients on day care so quickly and against their "better judgment." It was no simple matter to get the clinical staff to follow the research protocol. (Incidentally, the results of the study clearly indicated that it was far better for the average patient to have been placed on day care.)

It seems intuitively obvious that the naturalistic design—evaluating patients within the system as it actually operates—will yield a wealth of data that will help determine which programs are best for which kinds of patients. But, this is an assumption for which there is little, if any, evidence. It is, of course, true that one can evaluate treatment outcome in a naturalistic design. While information from such a study may be of value, its usefulness for determining differential effectiveness of alternative programs is severely limited for a number of reasons. Without the use of random assignment of patients to alternative treatment programs, it is highly unlikely that patients in two different programs are comparable. Therefore, any differences in average outcome of patients in the two programs may merely be a function of differences in initial patient characteristics that influence prognosis. In addition, without some control of the treatments being given, one cannot assume that the essential differences in the two treatment programs have been identified. For example, a comparison of a drug clinic program with an individual psychotherapy program would be of little value in indicating the superiority of either approach if one program also offered extensive social and vocational services while the other did not.

All Subjects versus Sampling

The second design issue is whether an attempt should be made to study all the subjects in a treatment program or to select samples. If the number of potential subjects involved in a program to be evaluated is small, then it may be quite feasible to study them all. However, if the number is large, it is unlikely that one can obtain data on all subjects without considerable sacrifice of accuracy or comprehensiveness of coverage. The precision with which national elections are predicted, based on extremely carefully selected, representative small samples, demonstrates the power of proper sampling. If sampling is employed, the hypothetical population being sampled should be the population for which both of the treatments being compared are considered reasonable, rather than all patients who are potentially available. For example, in a study of brief versus longer hospitalization (Herz, Endicott, and Spitzer 1975a,b), patients with certain diagnoses were excluded, such as those with chronic brain syndromes, since brief hospitalization for these conditions is usually inappropriate.

Routine Therapists' Ratings versus Special Therapists' Evaluations versus Independent Assessment Team

The last major design issue involves the evaluation of outcome. Should routinely collected data provided by the patients' therapists or special evaluations done by the patients' therapists be utilized, or should an independent assessment team conduct its own evaluation of the patient. There is naturally great appeal in using routinely completed therapists' ratings. The therapists presumably know the patients well and can see the patients without scheduling special evaluation sessions. They are required to complete certain records routinely and would not have to be paid extra for collecting such data.

The authors have had considerable experience using evaluation data collected by both therapists and independent assessors. In our experience, routinely collected data generally have low validity for research purposes (Endicott and Spitzer 1975; Endicott, Spitzer, and Fleiss 1975). Therapists lack motivation to give careful ratings, and usually have not been adequately trained to use the forms as they have been designed. In addition, because of frequent changes in therapists, the data usually come from a large number of different therapists; thus the sources of variance that lower reliability and validity are compounded.

The best data are obtained through the use of independent assessment teams that are specially trained. They not only overcome the motivational problems that plague therapists' ratings, but also provide ratings relatively uncontaminated by a desire to report good results or by any preconceptions regarding the differential effectiveness of the treatments being compared. Moreover, an independent assessment team's loyalty is to the evaluation project, and they do not resent collecting information on patient outcome, as therapists frequently do.

It is recognized that many projects cannot afford the luxury of an independent assessment team and are forced either to utilize data from therapists or to forgo evaluation of their therapeutic efforts. Given this restriction, the data should be collected as part of a special evaluation where the therapists know that the data will be used as part of a research project rather than just being stored in a computer for some vague purpose. The data so collected should be limited, if at all possible, to global judgments of severity of illness or improvement, or to information which is relatively objective and of clear relevance to the treatments being evaluated. Efforts to collect extensive data, such as comprehensive mental status evaluations from therapists, are doomed to failure for purposes of research evaluation. Furthermore, if therapists' data are to be used, some effort should be made to train them in the proper use of the evaluation procedures, to meet with them periodically to give them feedback on how the study is being conducted, and to review any procedural problems. In addition, the research staff should monitor the therapists' evaluations and return them for correction when necessary.

It is evident from the above discussion that we are proposing that optimal evaluation of differential effectiveness of treatment programs involve use of an experimental design, sampling based on specific inclusion and exclusion criteria, and the use of an independent assessment team for supplying outcome data. Unfortunately, the trend over the last decade has been in the opposite direction: the use of large information systems for studying ongoing services without an experimental design and the utilization of routinely collected data on all subjects supplied by the therapists. The failure of these systems to generate data of value for determining the differential effectiveness of different therapeutic approaches is striking and should lead users of these systems to explore alternative approaches.

Measures for Evaluation of Patient Outcome

There are three major types of criterion indices of patient improvement: status, psychopathology and social adjustment, and effect on others. Status involves such indices as whether the patient is in or out of the hospital or holding a job, percent of time spent in the community, and whether or not he/she is receiving public assistance. For some studies, such indices may, by themselves, give a clear indication of the superiority of a particular treatment approach. For example, in the study of brief hospitalization (Herz, Endicott, and Spitzer 1975a,b), it was shown that the two brief groups (with and without transitional day care) resumed their functioning in the community on a full-time basis more quickly than did a standard group, without a higher readmission rate.

There are many issues that need to be considered in the selection of an appropriate rating scale, because they differ from each other in a number of ways. In selecting or developing a rating scale for a particular purpose, the following should be considered: coverage, time period covered, who makes the ratings and how the data are collected, level of complexity of judgments required, how the judgments are recorded, time and ease of administration, level of experience and training required of personnel administering the procedure, how the data are summarized quantitatively, and, finally, the reliability and validity of the procedure. These issues have been discussed extensively in Spitzer and Endicott (1975).

Specific Rating Scales

The Psychiatric Status Schedule (PSS) (Spitzer et al. 1970) utilizes a structured interview schedule and an inventory of 321 items describing psychopathology and impaired role functioning (Figure 9-1). Since the PSS contains descriptions of small units of behavior and thus largely avoids the problem of scaling of severity, the interviewer who uses this form requires less clinical experience, although some training in making the judgments is needed. The items are summarized into seventeen factor-based scales of psychopathology and six scales of role functioning. These twenty-three measures can be further summarized into four factor-derived symptom scales and one scale of role functioning (Table 9-1). The data are collected during a 30- to 50-minute interview with the patient, and the specific items are dependent upon the responses given during the interview. Figure 9-2 demonstrates how these data can be used to evaluate the differential effectiveness of various treatment approaches.

The Psychiatric Evaluation Form (PEF) (Endicott and Spitzer 1972) utilizes an interview guide and accompanying 6-point rating scale of nineteen basic dimensions of psychopathology, five scales of role functioning, and one scale of overall severity of illness (Figure 9-3). These scales are further combined into five factor-derived summary scales of psychopathology and one summary scale of impaired role functioning. The rater is allowed to use all sources of information, such as clinical records, in addition to the interview of the patient. The interview guide allows the rater to limit the questions to those that are needed to make an adequate judgment of the broad dimensions under study without having to go into the detail needed for judging the kind of specific items that are in the PSS. Because the judgments are of levels of severity of specific dimensions of psychopathology, more clinical experience and exposure to patients is generally needed. Figure 9-4 demonstrates the use of the PEF scales in the evaluation of the differential effects of day and inpatient care.

Whereas the PSS and PEF describe the features of the patient's disturbance in terms of symptoms or symptom groupings (the multidimensional approach), the next technique described, the Global Assessment Scale (GAS), is used to assess the overall severity of the disturbance as a single dimension (Endicott et al. 1975). The multidimensional approach provides detailed information that is lost in a single overall measure. On the other hand, a measure of overall severity has the advantage of being a summary that allows a rater to combine the many elements of psychopathology into a single clinically meaningful index of severity of illness. In addition, in numerous studies of treatment efficacy, global ratings of status prove to be more sensitive to differential treatment effects than do measures of single dimensions of psychopathology (McGlashan 1973).

The GAS is a single rating scale for evaluating the overall functioning of a

INTERVIEW SCHEDULE	INVENTORY
How long does it take you to get dressed? (*Why does it take that long?*)	13. Indicates he spends an excessive amount of time dressing or grooming himself because of rituals, indecision, perfectionism, dawdling, or lethargy.

Mood

What kind of moods have you been in recently?	14. Says he has felt elated or "high" (do not include mere good spirits).

Worries

What kind of things do you worry about? If admits to worries: (*How much do you worry?*)	15. Mentions he worries a lot or that he can't stop worrying.

Fears

What kind of fears do you have? (*Are there things or situations you are afraid of?*) (*Anything else?*)	16. Admits to three or more different fears *or* says that he keeps feeling afraid of different things.
People sometimes have fears they know don't make sense—like crowds or certain activities. What kind of fears do you have like this?	17. Indicates he is fearful of losing his mind or losing control of his emotions.
If says he does not like or worries about an object or situation, ask: (*But are you afraid of ____?*)	18. Indicates a morbid fear that something terrible will happen to him.
	19. Indicates he has an irrational fear of a particular object or situation (e.g., crowds, heights) (phobia).
	20. Says he gets attacks of sudden fear or panic.
If indicates any fear: (*Does this fear of ____ prevent you from doing something you want to do?*)	21. Indicates his fear prevents him from participating in some activity

Anxiety

How often do you feel anxious or tense?
If unclear: *Nervous*
(*How much of the time do you feel this way?*)

22. Admits that he is often anxious.
23. Admits he feels anxious most of the time.

Restlessness

What about feeling restless?
If unclear: *Can't stay still*

24. Mentions he is often restless or is unable to stay still.

Depression

How often do you feel sad, depressed or blue?
(*How much of the time do you feel this way?*)

25. Admits he is often sad or depressed.
26. Admits he feels depressed most of the time.

Crying

When was the last time you felt like crying?

27. Admits he has felt like crying.

Self-appraisal

How do you feel about yourself?

28. Accuses himself of being unworthy, sinful, or evil.

Do you like yourself?
If unclear: (*When you compare yourself with other people, how do you come out?*)

29. Indicates he is bothered by feelings of inadequacy or that he doesn't like himself.

30. Indicates he is bothered by feelings of having done something terrible (guilt).

(*Do you feel that you are a particularly important person or that you have certain special powers or abilities?*)

31. In appraising himself he indicates an inflated view of his value or worth [grandiosity].

Figure 9-1. Page 2 of the Psychiatric Status Schedule.

Table 9-1. Basic Scoring System of the Second Edition of the Psychiatric Status Schedule

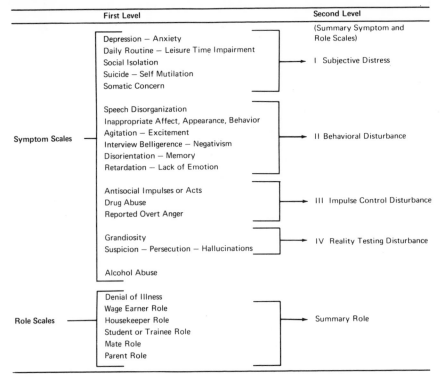

First Level		Second Level
		(Summary Symptom and Role Scales)
Symptom Scales	Depression — Anxiety Daily Routine — Leisure Time Impairment Social Isolation Suicide — Self Mutilation Somatic Concern	I Subjective Distress
	Speech Disorganization Inappropriate Affect, Appearance, Behavior Agitation — Excitement Interview Belligerence — Negativism Disorientation — Memory Retardation — Lack of Emotion	II Behavioral Disturbance
	Antisocial Impulses or Acts Drug Abuse Reported Overt Anger	III Impulse Control Disturbance
	Grandiosity Suspicion — Persecution — Hallucinations	IV Reality Testing Disturbance
	Alcohol Abuse	
Role Scales	Denial of Illness Wage Earner Role Housekeeper Role Student or Trainee Role Mate Role Parent Role	Summary Role

subject on a continuum, from psychological or psychiatric sickness to health during a specified time period (Figure 9-5). The time period that is assessed is generally the last week prior to an evaluation, although for special studies a longer time period may be more appropriate. The scale values range from 1, which represents the hypothetically sickest possible individual, to 100, the hypothetically healthiest. The scale is divided into ten equal intervals: 1-10, 11-20, and so on to 81-90 and 91-100. The defining characteristics of each 10-point interval comprise the scale. The two highest intervals, 81-90 and 91-100, are for those unusually fortunate individuals who not only are without significant psychopathology, but also exhibit many traits often referred to as positive mental health, such as superior functioning, a wide range of interests, social effectiveness, warmth, and integrity. The next interval, 71-80, is for individuals with no or only minimal psychopathology but who do not possess the positive mental health features noted above. Although some individuals rated above 70 may seek some form of assistance for psychological problems, the vast majority of individuals in treatment will be rated between 1 and 70. Most outpatients will be rated between 31 and 70, and most inpatients between 1 and

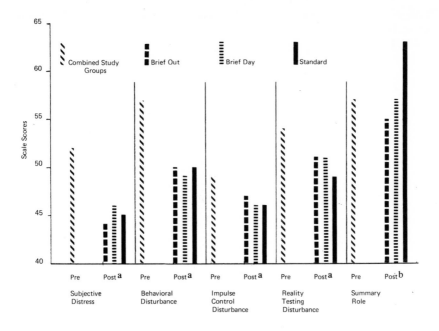

aDifferences in amount of improvement were not significant.

bDifferences in amount of improvement were significant at the 0.01 level.

Figure 9-2. Mean Psychiatric Status Schedule Scale Scores on Admission and at Three Weeks.

40. In determining a rating, one first selects the lowest interval which describes the subject's functioning during the preceding week. For example, a subject whose "behavior is considerably influenced by delusions" (range 21-30) should be given a rating in that range even though he/she has "marked impairment in several areas" (range 31-40). In order to determine the scale point within the 10-point interval, the defining characteristics of the two adjacent intervals are examined to determine whether the subject is closer to one or the other. For example, a subject in the range 21-30 who is much closer to the 11-30 range than the 31-40 range would be given a specific rating of 21, 22, or 23. A subject who seems to be equidistant from the two adjoining ranges is given a rating of 24, 25, 26, or 27. The value of the GAS for detecting changes is shown in Table 9-2.

Another instrument, the Family Evaluation Form (FEF) (Herz, Endicott, and Spitzer 1975b), is used to interview an informant about the patient and his/her family during the week prior to the evaluation. The FEF consists of an interview

INTERVIEW GUIDE

Original Complaint
If a psychiatric patient: Now I would like to hear about your problems or difficulties and how they led to your coming to the (hospital, clinic).

General Condition
Tell me how you have been feeling recently.
(*Anything else been bothering you?*)

Somatic Concerns
How is your physical condition?
Does any part of your body give you trouble?
Do you worry much about your health?
(If necessary, inquire for doctor's opinion about symptoms or illnesses.)

Appetite-Sleep-Fatigue
Disturbances in these areas are often associated with depression, anxiety, or somatic concerns.

What about your appetite for food?

Do you have any trouble sleeping or getting to sleep?
(*Why is that?*)
How easily do you get tired?

SCALES

Somatic Concerns
Excessive concern with bodily functions; preoccupation with one or more real or imagined physical complaints or disabilities; bizarre or unrealistic feelings or beliefs about his body or parts of body. Do not include mere dissatisfaction with appearance.

Anxiety and Depression

This section covers both Anxiety and Depression. The interviewer must determine to what extent the symptoms are associated with either one or the other or both dimensions.

What kinds of moods have you been in recently?

What kinds of things do you worry about? (*How much do you worry?*)

What kinds of fears do you have? (Any situations . . . activities . . . things?)

How often do you feel anxious or tense? (*When you are this way, do you react physically . . . like sweating, dizziness, cramps?*)

What about feeling restless?

How often do you feel sad, depressed, or blue?

When was the last time you felt like crying?

How do you feel about yourself? (*When you compare yourself with other people, how do you come out?*)

Is it hard for you to concentrate on things?

Do you enjoy things now as much as usual?

Anxiety
Remarks indicate feelings of apprehension, worry, anxiety, nervousness, tension, fearfulness, or panic. When clearly associated with any of these feelings, consider insomnia, restlessness, physical symptoms (e.g., palpitation, sweating, dizziness, cramps), or difficulty concentrating, etc.

Depression
Remarks indicate feelings of sadness, depression, worthlessness, failure, hopelessness, remorse, guilt, or loss. When clearly associated with any of these feelings, consider crying, insomnia, poor appetite, fatigue, loss of interest or enjoyment, difficulty concentrating, or brooding, etc.

Figure 9-3. Page 1 of the Psychiatric Evaluation Form.

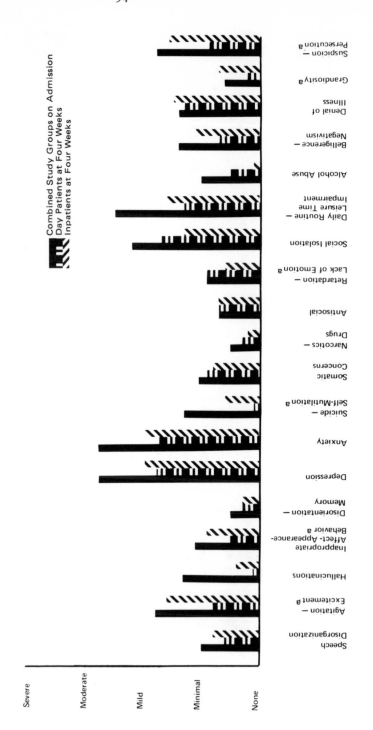

aDifference between day and inpatients significant at the 0.10 level.

Figure 9-4. Mean Psychiatric Evaluation Form Scale Scores for Study Groups on Admission and at Four-Week Follow-up.

Rate the subject's lowest level of functioning in the last week by selecting the lowest range which describes his function on a hypothetical continuum of mental health illness. For example, a subject whose "behavior is considerably influenced by delusions" (range 21-30) should be given a rating in that range even though he has "major impairment in several areas" (range 31-40). Use intermediary levels when appropriate (e.g., 35, 58, 63). Rate actual functioning independent of whether or not subject is receiving and may be helped by medication or some other form of treatment.

Name_____ ID No. _____ Consec. No. _____ Code. No. _____

Admission Date _____ Date of Rating _____ Rater _____ Rating _____

91-100 No symptoms, superior functioning in a wide range of activities, life's problems never seem to get out of hand, is sought out by others because of his warmth and integrity.

81-90 Transient symptoms may occur, but good functioning in all areas, interested and involved in a wide range of activities, socially effective, generally satisfied with life, "everyday" worries that only occasionally get out of hand.

71-80 Minimal symptoms may be present but no more than slight impairment in functioning, varying degrees of "everyday" worries and problems that sometimes get out of hand.

61-70 Some mild symptoms (e.g., depressive mood and mild insomnia) or some difficulty in several areas of functioning, but generally functioning pretty well, has some meaningful interpersonal relationships, and most untrained people would not consider him "sick."

51-60 Moderate symptoms or generally functioning with some difficulty (e.g., few friends and flat affect, depressed mood and pathological self-doubt, euphoric mood and pressure of speech, moderately severe antisocial behavior).

41-50 Any serious symptomatology or impairment in functioning that most clinicians would think obviously requires treatment or attention (e.g., suicidal preoccupation or gesture, severe obsessional rituals, frequent anxiety attacks, serious antisocial behavior, compulsive drinking).

31-40 Major impairment in several areas, such as work, family relations, judgment, thinking, or mood, or some impairment in reality testing or communication (e.g., speech is at times obscure, illogical or irrelevant), or single serious suicide attempt.

21-30 Unable to function in almost all areas (e.g., stays in bed all day) or behavior is considerably influenced by either delusions or hallucinations or serious impairment in communication (e.g., sometimes incoherent or unresponsive) or judgment (e.g., acts grossly inappropriately).

11-20 Needs some supervision to prevent hurting self or others, or to maintain minimal personal hygiene (e.g., repeated suicide attempts, frequently violent, manic excitement, smears feces), or gross impairment in communication (e.g., largely incoherent or mute).

1-10 Needs constant supervision for several days to prevent hurting self or others, or makes no attempt to maintain minimal personal hygiene.

Figure 9-5. Global Assessment Scale (GAS), by Robert L. Spitzer, M.D., Miriam Gibbon, M.S.W., Jean Endicott, Ph.D.

Table 9-2

Sensitivity to Change of Global Ratings of Overall Severity and Symptom Dimensions[a]

	Epsilon
Overall Severity	
GAS (Researchers)	0.83
GAS (Therapists)	0.75
PSS Total Score (Researchers)	0.75
FEF Total Score ($N = 58$)	0.67
MSER Overall Severity (Therapists)	0.47
Symptom Dimension	
PSS (Researchers)	
Subjective Distress	0.71
Behavioral Disturbance	0.49
Impulse Disorder	0.48
Reality Testing	0.47
Summary Role	0.36
MSER (Therapists)	
Depression Ideation–Mood	0.28
Suicide	0.55
Sleep–Appetite Disturbance	0.44
Somatic Concern	0.35
Anxiety	0.50
Inappropriate Appearance	0.37
Disorientation–Memory	0.09
Cognitive Disorganization	0.53
Hallucinations	0.45
Unusual Thoughts–Delusions	0.56
Suspiciousness	0.38
Anger–Negativism	0.33
Violence Ideation	0.43
Denial of Illness	0.06
Excitement	0.44
Retardation–Emotional Withdrawal	0.24
Alcohol Abuse	0.29
Drug Abuse	0.00
Judgment	0.43
Likeable	0.37

[a]N's vary from 102 to 107 except where otherwise noted.

guide and an inventory of 455 items. It takes approximately 45 minutes to complete. The items are grouped into 45 summary scales on the basis of content and similarity to factor-analytic studies of similar scales. Some of the items in the FEF describe the patient's psychopathology and are grouped into scales, such as Patient Subjective Distress or Patient Social Isolation. Other items describe psychopathology in family members and are grouped into scales describing family psychopathology and functioning. A third group of items has to with family difficulties that are "due to the patient." Whenever a family member's symptom or impaired functioning was acknowledged, the informant was asked, "Do you think it had anything to do with [the patient's] condition or was exacerbated by the patient's condition or situation?" These are grouped into scales such as Family Subjective Distress Due to the Patient. Other items reflect difficulties which directly involve the patient and reflect behaviors which have face validity, such as objective burdens on the family (i.e., has he/she hit anyone?). Figure 9-6 shows how two FEF measures of burden on the family were used in the study of brief hospitalization.

Considerable reliability and validity data are available on all four of these instruments. It has been demonstrated that two raters making joint observations of a series of patients will have a high degree of agreement, and that the scale scores can discriminate between groups known to differ on the relevant dimensions and can be used to evaluate improvement over time. They are discussed in more detail in previous papers (Spitzer et al. 1970; Endicott and Spitzer 1972; Herz, Endicott, and Spitzer 1975b).

There are many useful instruments for the evaluation of patient outcome, such as self-report measures—for example, the SCL-90 (Derogatis, Lipman, and Covi 1973)—which have not been discussed in this chapter. Other measures of social adjustment, such as the Social Adjustment Scale (Weissman 1975), and questionnaire measures completed by nonprofessional personnel, such as the recently developed Denver Community Mental Health Questionnaire (Ciarlo and Reihman 1974), also are promising.

Improvement is a complex, multifaceted process. It is unrealistic to expect that a single outcome measure will be sufficient for most studies. It has been found, in general, that measures of outcome often have a low and sometimes even negative intercorrelation. This suggests that multiple outcome measures are always desirable because they give a more complete picture of outcome from different points of view.

It is recognized that many of the suggestions mentioned seem complicated and difficult to implement in the average clinical setting. Inability to conduct a research study in an optimal fashion does not mean that it is thereafter better to do nothing than to do studies with limited outcome measures, degrees of control, etc. A great deal of useful information can be obtained from simple

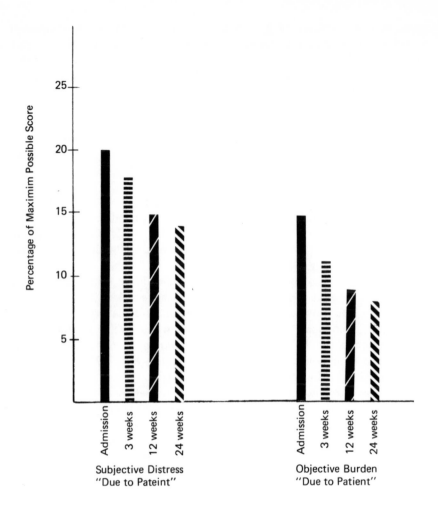

Figure 9-6. Change in Measures of Family Burden.

studies using gross measures, provided that the questions being answered are of relevance to decisions that have to be made regarding the best use of therapeutic resources. There is no substitute for a good idea.

References

Ciarlo, J.A., and Reihman, J. 1974. The Denver Community Mental Health Questionnaire: Development of a Multi-dimensional Program Evaluation Instrument. Unpublished manuscript.

Derogatis, L.R.; Lipman, R.S.; and Covi, L. 1973. "SCL-90: An Outpatient Psychiatric Rating Scale—Preliminary Report." *Psychopharmacological Bulletin* 9:13.

Endicott, J., and Spitzer, R.L. 1975. "Patient Assessment and Monitoring," in *Safeguarding Psychiatric Privacy—Computer Systems and Their Uses*, edited by E.M. Laska and R. Bank. New York: John Wiley & Sons, Inc.

_____, and _____. 1972. "What! Another Rating Scale? The Psychiatric Evaluation Form." *Journal of Nervous and Mental Disorders* 154:88-104.

_____, _____, and Fleiss, J.L. 1975. "Mental Status Examination Record (MSER): Reliability and Validity." *Comprehensive Psychiatry* 16:285-301.

_____, _____, _____, and Cohen, J. 1976. "The Global Assessment Scale: A Procedure for Measuring Overall Severity of Psychiatric Disturbance." *Archives of General Psychiatry.* In Press.

Herz, M.I.; Endicott, J.; and Spitzer, R.L. 1975a. "Brief Hospitalization of Patients with Families: Initial Results." *American Journal of Psychiatry* 132:413-418.

_____, _____, and _____. 1975b. "Brief versus Standard Hospitalization: The Families." Paper read at 128th annual meeting of the American Psychiatric Association, 5-9 May 1975, Anaheim, Calif.

_____, _____, _____, and Mesnikoff, A. 1971. "Day versus Inpatient Hospitalization: A Controlled Study." *American Journal of Psychiatry* 127:1371-1382.

Lyerly, S.B. 1973. *Handbook of Psychiatric Rating Scales*, 2d ed. National Institute of Mental Health, Bethesda, Md.

McGlashan, T., ed. 1973. *The Documentation of Clinical Psychotropic Drug Trials.* National Institute of Mental Health, Rockville, Md.

Spitzer, R.L., and Endicott, J. 1975. "Psychiatric Rating Scales in the Evaluation of Psychiatric Treatment," in *Comprehensive Textbook of Psychiatry*, edited by Friedman, A.M. and H.I. Kaplan. Baltimore: William and Wilkins Co.

_____, _____, Fleiss, J.L., and Cohen, J. 1970. "The Psychiatric Status Schedule: A Technique for Evaluating Psychopathology and Impairment in Role Functioning." *Archives of General Psychiatry* 23:41-55.

Weissman, M. 1975. "The Assessment of Social Adjustment." *Archives of General Psychiatry* 32:357-365.

10 Goal Attainment Scaling at a County Mental Health Service

Thomas J. Kiresuk

It began simply enough. Because our community mental health service was obliged to "do program evaluation," whatever that was, those of us involved decided that we might as well try to make it meaningful. Our thinking was that the information we collected in the name of program evaluation must be useful for management, ought to be useful scientifically, and might be useful to practitioners and patients. We might possibly capture some of the essence of the mental health enterprise, but certainly we would never explain, predict, and control it all. The madman in all of us—not to be confused with mental illness—would see to that.

The goal attainment method described here is only part of an evaluation effort that now has grown into a management-oriented system. Although this method could be used to evaluate just about anything, it was devised in a mental health setting and therefore relates to a special set of conceptual and measurement traditions. In particular, the method is addressed to one central question: how can one meet the requirements of program evaluation, a peculiar mixture of management and science, and at the same time provide for the unique characteristics of the treatment process and the aspirations of individual clients?

As of 1960, Hennepin County's Community Mental Health Service produced strictly descriptive and numerical reports in order to obtain funds from city, county, and state governments and to meet basic business and hospital accreditation standards. At that time, its program evaluation efforts consisted entirely of data related to the receipt and disbursement of funds, performance of certain activities, and some characteristics of patients. This was consonant with what Carstairs (1968) has labeled "evaluation of technic or process" and with the published report on the 1965 National Institute of Mental Health International Conference, which served to document the state of the art.

Goal Attainment Scaling was our solution to the problem of how to measure outcomes in the mental health enterprise—a diffuse, complex, evolving conglomerate of beliefs and activities that would not hold still for measurement. There were very many events and traditions, inside and outside psychology, that influenced the development of the measure. These are a few:

1. Under the direction of Stanley Cowle, county management and budgeting were evolving from efficiency-oriented management into a variety of planned program budgeting techniques and management by objectives. "Management by

objectives" can be considered an analogue to scientific theory building; the postulates of science and the ultimate corporate dedications of management can be considered the givens of self-evident truths to which all other laws must be related. In addition, both require ultimate empirical, objective, and (in the case of management science) pragmatic events to confirm the validity of the "theories." Outcome measures constitute the empirical base for the "theory" of an organization. The coincidental development of this style of management locally, along with the pressure for empirical evidence for treatment effectiveness and for support of theories of mental illness, strongly influenced the general nature of the outcome measure.

2. The schools of motivation and dynamic psychology indicate that the human organism is trying to "get at" something. Knowing what that something is and studying the means by which it is attempted or attained constitute a central issue for measurement. Level-of-aspiration studies by Lewin et al. (1965), for instance, compare actual performance of a subject to hoped-for expectations. Achievement motivation studies also lead to examination of goals and their measurement. In their study of the motivation of economic achievement, McClelland and Winter (1969) developed a goal attainment measure to determine progress toward a set of goals that is uniquely determined for each subject.

3. In experimental psychology, the work of Skinner (1953) has led to the development of behavior therapies in mental health settings. As pointed out by Ullman and Krasmer (1965), these behavior therapies require careful documentation of current behavior and specifications of the behavioral change to be achieved by treatment. A natural extension of this procedure would be to list these behavioral goals in a goal attainment format.

4. Pollard and Mitchell (1972), in their article on decision theory and power, state that a common theme in a number of areas of psychology is that "behavior is a function of the probability or degree to which behavior leads to various outcomes or consequences and the value of utility of these consequences." Our measure requires setting expected levels of outcome. In order to do so, one has to guess what the patient is going to be like or the patient has to foresee what he/she wants to be like, as a result of treatment. Subjective probability—individual judgment of the likelihood that an outcome will occur as the result of an action—is a major construct in decision theories and is the process required to construct a range of alternatives for each goal dimension.

5. In the history of psychological measurement, there is a central ideological conflict. Those of the "idiographic" point of view hold that the individual's personality is to be understood and measured only in terms of himself/herself—the unique constellation of individual history, behaviors, values, and other attributes—and that general measures across all persons would not capture the essence of each individual. On the other hand, those of the "nomothetic" point of view stress the development of general laws of personality—that individual characteristics can be applied to general populations of individuals. Related to

this measurement issue, Kiesler (1966) has labeled assumptions of patient uniformity and therapist uniformity as fallacies in the field of therapy research. The question remains, however: How far can one go toward recognizing the uniqueness of the individual before one destroys all possibility of formulating general principles? Therapy research is only one corner of the mental health program evaluation enterprise, but both traditions, idiographic and nomothetic, must be honored in order to carry out a total evaluation.

6. Finally, a very important tradition may be termed the philosophy of mental health. Schofield (1967), among others, has discussed the fact that value systems of individuals and of society to a large extent determine the definitions of mental health. Ultimately, management and clinical goals are derivatives of these value systems. This is easiest to see on the clinical level. Currently, it is a patient's luck of the draw that determines whether one's therapist will strive to save the marriage or facilitate its dissolution; help obtain an abortion or try to prevent it; or consider homosexuality a sin, a symptom of schizophrenia, or a problem of social adjustment. This relativism pervades all levels of the mental health enterprise, and outcome measurement has to deal with this issue. An excerpt from Alexander Solzhenitsyn's Nobel Prize acceptance speech, although not addressed to the field of mental health, nevertheless summarizes the raw stuff of outcome determination:

There are at least several scales of values in the world: one for evaluating events near at hand, another for events far away; aging societies possess one, young societies another; successful people one, unsuccessful yet another. The divergent scales of values scream in discordance, they dazzle and daze us, and to avoid the pain, we wave aside all other values but our own.

Tailoring a Goal Attainment System to the Setting

The Hennepin County Mental Health Service is located in a downtown public general hospital, less than a mile from the state university. When we began our evaluation project, the mental health service consisted of approximately 100 employees who served 5,000 patients and other clients per year. The service had these subunits: inpatient, outpatient, day hospital, child care, medication maintenance, social rehabilitation, and consultation and education. Since then a crisis intervention unit has been added. The treatment staff included psychiatrists, psychologists, social workers, nurses, allied health specialists, and students of all disciplines. Treatment philosophies and corresponding definitions of mental health varied accordingly. The patients were of all ages and diagnostic categories, of both sexes from both the middle and lower socioeconomic status levels. The case load included university students as well as the uneducated.

Typical of the 1960s, the mental health service existed in an uncertain administrative climate in which the role of mental institutions, the balance between traditional and community-oriented services, and the roles of the various professions and of the consumer were all being reassessed. Concurrent with this challenge to existing concepts, values, and activities, the groundwork for future patterns of human-service care was being established.

Because a management information system of sorts existed, the immediate issue was that of devising a measure or set of measures to determine effectiveness of our services. It was our hope that this measure (or more likely, a test battery) already existed. The measure would have to satisfy the usual standards of psychological measurement, be meaningful to therapists, be useful in research, meet administrative needs, be capable of numerical relationship to process measures and resource allocation, be comprehensible to patients and consumer representatives, and be related to rational management and scientific inquiry while retaining the sweet mystery of life.

There is no such measure, of course. In that sentence resides four years of correspondence, literature reviews, site visits, file drawers full of evaluation systems used by others, and several registries of questionnaire items, stabled and stillborn.

Because we could not find or devise fixed standards of mental health to apply to all patients and therapists, we set no limitations on content. Turning to the administrator, therapist, and patient, we in effect said, "You tell us what you are trying to do, and we will help you measure progress toward that event or entity, whatever it is. Use anyone's standards or tests; make up new ones if you like. Pick outcome events so that they will be indicators of the essential quality you are after, even if you can't state exactly what that quality is. Tailor these dimensions and outcomes for each program or individual. If they are truly unique to that patient, you need never use them again. If common dimensions and outcomes start to occur for particular kinds of patients or setting, group them. You can combine commonly used scales or dimensions with unique, used-only-once scales. If you think you know best and have the power to enforce your judgment, just write down your standards, as indicated above, and you will find out how well these standards have been met."

Essentially, then, the method was set up to have the following characteristics: (1) a set of dimensions devised for or by the individual; (2) a system to assign weights among the dimensions; (3) a set of expected outcomes devised for each outcome; (4) a follow-up scoring of these outcomes; and (5) a score summarizing the outcome across all the dimensions.

Figure 10-1 illustrates a sample follow-up guide. Five scale headings were chosen by the clinician as being important concerns. The titles were chosen for the scales to help the follow-up worker understand the nature of the dimension on which the patient was being assessed. Outcome levels were then selected for some scales with the patient's involvement; others were selected by the clinician alone. The expected level with treatment on the first scale was tailor-made for this patient, and indicated that some practical steps would be taken by the patient, but they would be taken with some ambivalence. The range of outcomes on either side of this expected outcome was also tailor-made, and was within the capacity of this patient. The reasoning behind the outcome selection went as follows: given this patient, with a specific background, environment, defined abilities and liabilities and hopes for the future, given the capabilities of our treatment staff to treat such cases, as well as the current state of knowledge, what can we expect the patient to be doing, to be like, at the time of follow-up?

Because the scales were weighted relative to one another, any set of values could be used. The check marks indicated the clinician's estimate of the level at intake. The asterisks indicated the scoring by the follow-up worker. Using the formula derived by Robert Sherman, a T score summarized the outcome for this patient. Comparing the intake with the follow-up score provided a difference score, or estimate of change during treatment.

Implementation of the System

Once developed, the technique appeared to be straightforward, but basic questions remained about its use. The National Institute of Mental Health sponsored a Program Evaluation Project in 1969 to determine the characteristics of the measure, to run treatment comparisons in the outpatient unit of the center, and to disseminate the method and findings. Some of the questions about the measure were: Would anyone use it? Who? In what settings? If it were used, what would be the content of the scales, how reliable would the method be, would it make a difference who constructed the follow-up guide, how would it relate to other measures, and what would be the characteristics of the score? What could the measure be used for, and would it make any difference?

To answer these questions, the following studies were undertaken:

1. Comparisons of group, individual, day hospital, or medication treatment.
2. Comparisons between professional disciplines and between students and staff.
3. Comparisons of Valium and placebo, with or without individual psychotherapy.
4. Comparison of Goal Attainment Scaling with the MMPI, Brief Psychiatric Rating Scale, Self-Rating Symptom Scale, Taylor Manifest Anxiety Scale, and Consumer Satisfaction Scale.
5. Study of selected population and problem groups.
6. Study of the accuracy of clinician's expectations.

The investigative method employed by the project was complex, but included these features:

1. A follow-up guide was constructed by an intake worker after one of two interviews with the patient.

Level at Intake: ✓

Level at Follow-up: *

Level at Intake: 29.4
Goal Attainment Score (Level at Follow-up): 62.2
Goal Attainment Change Score: +32.8

Sample Clinical Guide: Crisis Intervention Center

PROGRAM EVALUATION PROJECT

GOAL ATTAINMENT FOLLOW-UP GUIDE

	SCALE HEADINGS AND SCALE WEIGHTS				
Check whether or not the scale has been mutually negotiated between patient and CIC interviewer. SCALE ATTAINMENT LEVELS	Yes X No — SCALE 1: Education ($w^1 = 20$)	Yes No X — SCALE 2: Suicide ($w^2 = 30$)	Yes No X — SCALE 3: Manipulation ($w^3 = 25$)	Yes X No — SCALE 4: Drug Abuse ($w^4 = 30$)	Yes X No — SCALE 5: Dependency on CIC ($w^5 = 10$)
a. Most unfavorable treatment outcome thought likely (−2)	Patient has made no attempt to enroll in high school. ✓	Patient has committed suicide.	Patient makes rounds of community service agencies demanding medication, and refuses other forms of treatment. ✓	Patient reports addiction to "hard narcotics" (heroin, morphine).	Patient has contacted CIC by telephone or in person at least seven times since his first visit.
b. Less than expected success with treatment (−1)	Patient has enrolled in high school, but at time of follow-up has dropped out.	Patient has acted on at least one suicidal impulse since her/his first contact with the CIC, but has not succeeded. ✓	Patient no longer visits CIC with demands for medication but continues with other community agencies and still refuses other forms of treatment. ✓	Patient has used "hard narcotics," but is not addicted, and/or uses hallucinogens (LSD, pot) more than four times a month. ✓	Patient has contacted CIC 5-6 times since intake. ✓

c. Expected level of treatment success (0)	Patient has enrolled, and is in school at follow-up, but is attending class sporadically (misses an average of more than a third of classes during a week). *	Patient reports she/he has had at least four suicidal impulses since her/his first contact with the CIC but has not acted on any of them.	Patient no longer attempts to manipulate for drugs at community service agencies, but will not accept another form of treatment.	Patient has not used "hard narcotics" during follow-up period, and uses hallucinogens between 1 and 4 times a month. *	Patient has contacted CIC 3 to 4 times since intake.
d. More than expected success with treatment (+1)	Patient has enrolled, is in school at follow-up, and is attending classes consistently, but has no vocational goals. *		Patient accepts non-medication treatment at some community agency. *	Patient uses hallucinogens less than once a month.	
e. Best anticipated success with treatment (+2)	Patient has enrolled, is in school at follow-up, is attending classes consistently, and has some vocational goal.	Patient reports she/he has had no suicidal impulses since her/his first contact with the CIC.	Patient accepts non-medication treatment, and by own report shows signs of improvement.	At time of follow-up, patient is not using any illegal drugs.	Patient has not contacted CIC since intake. *

Figure 10-1. Sample Goal Attainment Follow-up Guide from Kiresuk Monograph Article.

2. The patient was randomly assigned to treatment when appropriate.
3. The therapist and patient did not know the content of the follow-up guide.
4. The follow-up guide was scored by a follow-up worker who was not part of the mental health service staff. The follow-up worker also obtained a consumer satisfaction report.

As there were no restrictions on content of the scales, the project also wanted to discover what clinicians produced as indicators of therapy progress. To this end, Garwick and Lampman (1972) have completed content and quantitative analyses of project data and isolated a set of content areas that summarize the general areas used by the mental health service staff.

Management applications have included follow-up guides for administrative units (Figure 10-2), a study on the effects of feedback to therapists on subsequent outcome scores, and outcome of treatment as it relates to method of intake. Standard scales are under development, as are methods of relating scale content and scale outcome to management goals, related cost estimates, and the problem-oriented record system described by Weed (1969).

After three years of the four-year project, some findings relate to the questions already listed. In the outpatient unit 2,500 follow-up guides have been constructed, averaging about four scales each; 900 follow-up interviews have been held. The Goal Attainment Score has a roughly symmetrical distribution (Figure 10-3), with a mean of 50.00, a standard deviation of 10, and a range of 20 to 80. Various agreement indices are currently being determined, using a total of 170 patients. The correlation between outcome scores on two follow-up guides constructed independently by different staff at different times for the same client is approximately 0.70. Content analyses of these two sets of follow-up guides indicate substantial content agreement, a correlation of 0.88. Agreement between follow-up workers, independently scoring the same guides at different times, with an average of 26 days between scorings, is also about 0.70.

In their study, Garwick and Lampman have found twenty scale headings that can probably include or subsume most of the content of scales (Figure 10-4). These include aggression, alcohol use, anxiety, and psychopathological symptoms. These content areas are just about what one would expect, given this kind of staff and setting, although until now no one knew for certain what the objectives of our clinical operation would be.

Potential Applications

In developing about 3,000 contacts with other locations, we have received valuable criticism and suggestions, as well as new ideas for applications that probably would not have occurred to us. There are well over 150 users and former users of Goal Attainment Scaling, and others are in various stages of conducting formal and informal studies.

Scale Attainment Levels	Scale (1): Assumption of Suicide Telephone Responsibilities	Scale (2): Implementation of Clinical Evaluation of Services	Scale (3): Patient Satisfaction with the Crisis Intervention Center
Most Unfavorable Outcome Thought Likely	Crisis Unit is unable to handle all incoming suicide calls.		Patient satisfaction is not systematically sampled by the Crisis Intervention Center, or a format for doing so has been devised but not implemented. *
Less Than Expected Programmatic Success	Crisis Unit is able to handle all incoming suicide calls but is unable to implement improvements, such as the use of multiple phones.	Planning phase is completed to assess alternative research designs for clinical evaluation of the Crisis Intervention Center's services (i.e., various forms of Goal Attainment Scaling are assessed).	Questionnaire format for assessing patient satisfaction is formulated or implemented on a sampling basis. Less than 40% of the patients sampled indicate satisfaction.
Expected Programmatic Success	Crisis Unit assumes total responsibility for the Suicide Service, and improves service by implementing multiple phones, integrating contacts into uniform crisis records, etc.	Planning phase is completed, and a decision has been made on most appropriate method of evaluation; implementation has begun.	Patient satisfaction questionnaire is implemented, and 40 to 60% indicate satisfaction.
More Than Expected Programmatic Success	In addition to the "Expected Level of Success," the Crisis Unit routinely follows up on suicide contacts (follow-ups may be defined as contacting the caller or his "significant others," checking with referral agency if a referral has been made, etc.) *	Evaluation methodology has been chosen and has been in operation for at least six months.	Patient satisfaction questionnaire is implemented, and 61 to 80% indicate satisfaction.
Best Anticipated Programmatic Success		In addition to "More Than Expected Level of Success," data are used by Unit Director for policymaking, and/ or feedback of results to staff has begun. *	Patient satisfaction questionnaire is implemented, and more than 80% indicate satisfaction.

*Level of Follow-up.

Figure 10-2. Sample Administrative Follow-up Guide, Crisis Intervention Center.

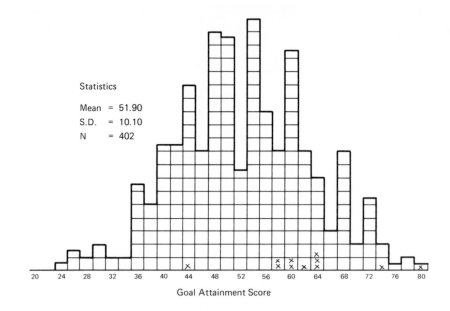

The X's indicate the distribution of one therapist's Goal Attainment Scores.

Figure 10-3. Hennepin County Mental Health Services: Distribution of Goal Attainment Scores for the First 402 Patients Followed-up.

Some questions being investigated are particularly intriguing. One such question is: Who should and who can set the goals? To this end, population groups on which the method is being tested in various settings include disturbed children, delinquent youths, adult prisoners and parolees, adult outpatients, the aged, and graduate students.

Other questions being asked in several locations include: What are the expectations of professionals for various population groups, and what are the expectations of individuals within these groups for themselves? How accurate are these expectations? What effect on outcome do these expectations have? And, if a patient devises her/his own treatment goals and goal indicators, what effect does this have on the outcome of her/his treatment? (We are studying this last question in our day treatment unit, using a special Goal Attainment Scaling form developed by Geoffrey Garwick.)

All this work is new and exciting, involving considerable ingenuity. Not all of it, however, has been around long enough to have received the kind of cautious, thorough, critical peer review that is necessary to understand the work in the context of psychological measurement and to determine the optimal applications that can be made.

		FOLLOW-UP GUIDES INCLUDING PHRASES	
GROUPINGS OF THE ISOLATED PHRASES		N	Percent
Work:	Job, vocation, employment, performance, etc.	49	18.1
Relationships:	People, social activities, live alone, friends, etc.	47	17.4
Anxiety-Depression:	Depression, tension, "the blues," fear, stress, etc.	30	11.1
Family-Marital:	Children, in-laws, wife, husband, marriage, etc.	28	10.4
Self-definition:	Self-control, decisions, responsibility, etc.	27	10.0
Treatment:	Hospitalization, treatment, medication, therapy, etc.	22	8.1
Sexuality:	Sexual intercourse, dates, masturbation, homosexuality, etc.	17	6.3
Suicide:	Self-destruction, suicidal impulses, self-mutilation, etc.	12	4.4
Education:	School, grades, attendance, graduation, college, etc.	8	3.0
Physical Complaints:	Sleeping, tics, chest pains, poor appetite, ulcers, etc.	4	1.5
Miscellaneous:		26	9.6
Total		270	100.0

Figure 10-4. Problem Categories Mentioned on Goal Attainment Follow-up Guides of 270 Randomly Selected Hennepin County Mental Health Service Outpatients.

To many potential users, for example, the openness of the method may be somewhat baffling. This is because Goal Attainment Scaling is not a scale with fixed content and standardized administration. Any objective content may be used to judge progress toward any goals. The content need not be the goals themselves, but indicators of goal achievement. Those organizations having patients and cultures in common can exchange content lists, develop their own local norms, or develop shared norms. If patient and staff composition is fairly constant, a standard language can be devised (and apparently has been in one setting). The reliabilities will vary with the usage: the content, the rigor with which outcomes are specified, the choice of follow-up dates, the nature of the follow-up workers and goal creators, and so forth.

The score itself has been an issue for some potential users. Some prefer that numbers other than zero stand for the expected level, such as a positive integer (with positive implications) or something that fits their intuitive feeling for numbers. Others prefer a number other than 50 to be the central T-score value, such as 70 (for passing) or 100, as in I.Q. scores. Some prefer that the -2 should be at the bottom of the sheet, and so on. Adjustments to the method depend on what you want to do. In many cases no number at all need be used; simple inspection might be sufficient. Basically, the formula takes into account varying numbers of scales and weights in producing a score that has equal importance for each patient in a sample of patients.

If one is looking for differences in a formal study, the formula is designed to help find such differences with a slightly smaller sample. There is some value in selecting procedures that have been used by others, primarily in order to be able to relate one's findings to theirs, perhaps taking advantage of norms and measurement characteristics that have already been developed.

The costs also depend on what one wants to do. If you want to check the accuracy of your own expectations or the outcomes of your clients, it costs practically nothing in terms of equipment or personnel: about 20 minutes to write a guide and probably another 20 minutes to do a telephone follow-up (if you don't use a volunteer). If you want to perform treatment comparisons, the costs depend on the design, method, sample size, type of analysis, and questions to be answered. If you want to do both management and clinical follow-up guides, continuously modify the program and its objectives according to the results; then the outpatient model developed by Dean Beaulieu, Robert Walker, James Baxter, and the staff in the Hennepin County outpatient unit might provide a good estimate. It amounts to one senior clerk and one evaluation technician to take care of the chores and do quality-control checks in a unit seeing 2,000 patients per year. This model integrates outcome benefit measures with administrative process measures.

Evaluation of the System

Generally, the advantage of the method lies in its flexible structure, its ability to accommodate a wide variety of measures. A presumed advantage is that the method requires that each patient be measured only on dimensions that are believed to be specifically relevant. Another presumed advantage is that only the meaningful range of values within a dimension is chosen, and unlikely extremes are not retained. And finally, particular, objectively determinable outcomes that one selects in advance permit an audit of the goal setting and perhaps help reduce some of the subjective rater bias involved in global ratings.

The difficulties in using the method relate to its novel aspects. It takes a while to get some people to think in terms of objective outcomes. Also, because of the relativistic framework, comparisons across patient populations and repeated measures over time require additional appraisal of the goals and their outcomes according to the particular value system and standards of the new frame of reference. Technical solutions for this dilemma are planned, some nearly completed, but every effort to escape the ultimate relativism has so far resulted in only another variety of relativism. Whatever the perspective, including the national viewpoint, the resulting standards always appear to be just another follow-up guide, determined for a particular era and society.

What place does the measure have in total program evaluation systems? With regard to this larger question, whatever the final definition of mental health will be, it appears that it will include combinations of physical, social, psychological, and interpersonal problems along with the interpretation of these problems by a variety of individuals and organizations. It appears that locally we are moving toward a program evaluation system that will provide a rational, coherent, and logically consistent explanatory and descriptive network of narrative and quantitative statements. These statements will take into account the definitions and efficiency of its activities. It will use management and evaluation data to influence subsequent goal setting and goal attainment in a continuous feedback process.

This evaluation system, of course, will also be another crystal palace of rational enlightenment—the best that reason, science, and government operation can devise at the time. The question is: To what extent can this system accommodate the not-so-rational facts of life (that we all know about)? For instance, how do we accommodate the "underground man" of Dostoevski's *Notes from the Underground*? How can we take account of the well-known potential of managers to choose nonoptimal decision theory alternatives, to go counter to the rational structures they themselves promulgate? What will happen if the staff and clients encounter William Barrett's irrational man in themselves? To what extent can we expect that individuals will speak their unspeakable goals, that the system will be more than a superficial, rational-appearing structure that we leave when we get down to the real business of living?

Suppose the ultimate postulates of mental health management emerge as the credo: "I believe in determinism, pragmatism, materialism, humanism, psychological hedonism, tranquility, and, when compatible with these, the reduction of human suffering. The problems of all those entering this microcosm will be interpreted and corrected according to these principles." Then I believe we will be unable to answer existential therapist R.D. Laing and the others who tell us that such a credo forces the individual to become what he/she is not, to adopt the prescribed roles of the patient in the mental health scenario.

In mental health one must sooner or later deal with ultimate values of living: those of the client, staff, and the organization. To be sure, the Goal Attainment Scaling method is only one way to attempt to accommodate those values. Yet in constructing our goal attainment model we sought to make room for both life strategies—that of management, seeking to devise a sensible, pragmatic system, and that of the individual, mentally ill or not, searching for what Lionel Trilling called the expression of authentic self.

References

Barrett, W. 1962. *Irrational Man.* Garden City: Doubleday Anchor Books.

Beaulieu, D., and Baxter, J. 1972. "Hennepin County Adult Outpatient Evaluation Program." Unpublished report, Minneapolis: Program Evaluation Project.

Carstairs, G. 1968. "Problems of Evaluation Research," in *Community Mental Health: An International Perspective*, edited by R.H. Williams and L.D. Ozarin. San Francisco: Jossey-Bass.

Colby, K. 1964. "Psychotherapeutic Process." *Annual Review of Psychology* 15:347-370.

Cowle, S. 1971. "Planning Programming Budgeting System." Minneapolis: Office of the County Administrator, Hennepin County.

_____ . 1972. "Hennepin County Program Budgeting." Minneapolis: Office of the County Administrator, Hennepin County.

Drucker, P. 1964. *Managing for Results.* New York: Harper and Row.

Feigl, H., and Sellars, W. (eds.). 1949. *Readings in Philosophical Analysis.* New York: Appleton-Crofts, Inc.

Garwick, G. 1973. "Guide to Goals I." Unpublished report. Minneapolis: Program Evaluation Project.

_____ , and Lampman, S. 1972. "Typical Problems Bringing Patients to a Community Mental Health Center." *Community Mental Health Journal* 8:271-280.

Kiesler, D.J. 1966. "Some Myths of Psychological Research and the Search for a Paradigm." *Psychological Bulletin* 65:110-136.

Kiresuk, T.J., and Sherman, R.E. 1968. "Goal Attainment Scaling: A General Method for Evaluating Comprehensive Community Mental Health Programs." *Community Mental Health Journal* 4:443-453.

Laing, R.D. 1969. *The Divided Self.* New York: Pantheon Books.

Lewin, K.; Dembo, T.; Festinger, L.; and Sears, P. 1965. "Level of Aspiration," in *Personality and the Behavior Disorders*, edited by J. McV. Hunt. New York: Roland Press.

McClelland, D.C., and Winter, D.G. 1969. *Motivating Economic Achievement.* New York: Free Press.

Pollard, W.E., and Mitchell, T.R. 1972. "Decision Theory Analysis of Social Power." *Psychological Bulletin* 78:433-446.

Schofield, W. 1967. *Psychotherapy: The Purchase of Friendship.* Englewood Cliffs, N.J.: Prentice-Hall, Inc.

Skinner, B.F. 1953. *Science and Human Behavior.* New York: Macmillan Co.

Stelmachers, Z.; Lund, S.; and Meade, C. 1972. "Hennepin County Crisis Intervention Center: Evaluation of Its Effectiveness." *Evaluation* 1:61-65.

Trilling, L. 1972. *Sincerity and Authenticity.* Cambridge, Mass.: Harvard University Press.

Ullman, L.P., and Krasmer, L. 1965. *Case Studies in Behavior Modification.* New York: Holt, Reinhart and Winston, Inc.

Walker, R.A. 1972. "The Ninth Panacea: Program Evaluation." *Evaluation* 1:45.

Weed, L.L. 1969. *Medical Records, Medical Examination and Patient Care.* Cleveland: Case Western Reserve University Press.

11 A Decision-Theoretic Approach to the Evaluation of Community Mental Health Centers

Marcia Guttentag

Accountability is the key term during times of economic hardship, when social programs must fight for the monies needed to stay alive. The birth of many new and innovative social programs marked the affluent 1960s. Many of these programs are facing death in the fiscal distress of the 1970s. The social programs that survive this struggle for resources will have to be accountable.

But, accountable to whom? The move for accountability can be seen as many social programs begin to more seriously define their audiences—the people affected by them—and the decisionmakers who are important to their survival. The Community Mental Health Centers (CMHCs) have a clear advantage because they are community-based and community-oriented programs and have realized from the start that citizen representation in catchment areas is a necessary part of the peer review process. Furthermore, CMHC planners have dealt with the peer review aspects of both the planning and evaluation of services from the very initiation of their programs. Thus, the question of their accountability is reasonably clear. The next step in CMHC evaluation is to develop conceptual frameworks and methodologies that may be built into both the peer review process and citizen participation, as integral parts of planning and evaluation. For this, an evaluation paradigm is needed that will formally integrate the peer review process in the planning of services to be offered and the aspects of these services that will be evaluated. But how can citizen input be used? After all, citizens are not professionally trained. How can they know what to plan for and what to evaluate?

A useable evaluation paradigm must separate the specification of goals from the technical planning and evaluation of programs. Such a paradigm should permit citizens to indicate what their values and overall goals are for community mental health programs. Professionals then can formulate the content of services that they believe will meet these objectives. Thus, evaluation is the determination of the extent to which these citizen-generated goals are being met.

An appropriate evaluation paradigm for CMHCs must also meet the following important requirements:

1. *Multiple measurement.* Since the goals of any CMHC program are always complex and multiple, a useful evaluation paradigm must have multiple measure requirements built into it—requirements not added at the discretion of the researcher.

2. *Data inclusiveness.* All forms of measurement are expensive. It is therefore essential that in CMHC evaluation, no data be thrown out or omitted because they do not meet the exacting standards of classical statistical tests. A useful evaluation paradigm for CMHCs should be data inclusive, i.e., observational data, formal measurement, archival data, etc., should be used when available. The extent to which hypotheses can be revised will vary according to the diagnosticity of the data. (Diagnosticity relates to reliability, validity, etc.). In addition, the evaluation paradigm should permit the integration of widely varying types of data with the values and goals generated by the peer review, so that progress toward these goals may be evaluated.

3. *Relating CMHC programs to catchment demographic characteristics and needs.* An evaluation paradigm for CMHCs must also permit an integration of data on the demography of catchment areas with data on program effectiveness. Such a paradigm should therefore be able to combine data generated through social area analysis methods with program effectiveness data.

4. *Continuous feedback.* Continuous or intermittent feedback should be an integral part of the evaluation paradigm. Relevant data should be available whenever decisions must be made.

The decision-theoretic (multiattribute utility) and Bayesian statistical evaluation paradigm meet the criteria that have been enumerated.

In the following sections, a simple multiattribute utility procedure (Edwards, Guttentag, and Snapper 1975) will be described, followed by (1) an illustration of the application of this approach, and (2) the use of Bayesian statistics in data integration.

The MAUT Evaluation Paradigm

The MAUT Evaluation Paradigm which follows was adapted from Edwards (1971). It is oriented toward easy communication and use in environments in which time is short and decisionmakers are multiple. It is a method that is psychologically meaningful to decisionmakers who are required to render judgments which are intuitively reasonable.

The essence of any multiattribute utility measurement is that each outcome to be evaluated is located on each dimension of value by a procedure that may consist of experimentation, naturalistic observation, judgment, or some combination of these. These location measures are combined by means of an aggregation rule, usually a simple, weighted linear combination. The weights are numbers describing the importance of each dimension of value relative to the others. The numbers are judgmentally obtained.

The procedure consists of ten steps:

Step 1. Identify the person or organization whose utilities are to be maximized. If, as is often the case, several organizations have an interest and input in the decision, they must all be identified and induced to cooperate. This is the beginning of the implementation of the peer review process required for CMHC evaluation.

Step 2. Identify the issue or issues (i.e., decisions) to which the utilities are relevant. The same CMHC programs may have many different values, depending on context and purpose. In general, utility is a function of (1) the evaluator, (2) the entity being evaluated, and (3) the purpose for which the evaluation is being made.

Step 3. Identify the programs to be evaluated. These include not only all current programs but also any conceivable action alternative—tried or untried.

Step 4. Identify the relevant dimensions of value. The number of relevant dimensions of value should be kept down, for reasons that shortly will become apparent. This can often be done by restating and combining goals, or by moving upward in a goal hierarchy, thereby using fewer, more general values. Even more important, it can be done by simply omitting the less important goals. There is no requirement that the list evolved in this step be complete. Pragmatically, these values can be elicited from peer review groups under consensus rules, or from individuals privately.

Step 5. Rank the dimensions in order of importance. This ranking job, like Step 4, can be performed by an individual, by representatives of conflicting interests acting separately, or by those representatives acting as a group. One preferred technique is the group processes method. This method allows the participants to start from a common information base and to air all arguments. Each individual then proffers separate judgments.

Step 6. Rate dimensions in importance, preserving ratios. The rating is accomplished by assigning the least important dimension an importance of 10. (10 is used rather than 1 to permit subsequent judgments to be finely graded in integers.) The next least-important dimension is then considered. How many times more important (if any) is it than the least important? A number is then assigned that reflects that ratio. As each new judgment is made, the list is checked and a set of implied ratios is formed. Thus, if a dimension is assigned a weight of 20, while another is assigned a weight of 80, the 20 dimension is one-fourth as important as the 80 dimension. When the most important dimensions are assigned, there will be many checks to perform. Typically, respondents will want to revise previous judgments to make them consistent with present ones. Individual differences are likely to arise.

Step 7. Sum the importance weights, divide each by the sum, and multiply by 100. This is a purely computational step which converts importance weights into numbers that, mathematically, are rather like probabilities. The choice of a 0-to-100 scale is, of course, purely arbitrary.

At this step, the folly of including too many dimensions at Step 4 becomes glaringly apparent. If 100 points are to be distributed over a set of dimensions and some dimensions are much more important than others, then the less important dimensions will have nontrivial weights only if there are not too many of them. In general, eight dimensions are sufficient, and fifteen is too many. In view of this, respondents should be discouraged at Step 4 from being too finely analytical. Moreover, it may occur that the list of dimensions will be revised later, and that revision, if it occurs, will typically consist of including more rather than fewer.

Step 8. Measure the location of each entity being evaluated on each dimension. The word "measure" is used rather loosely here. There are three classes of dimensions: purely subjective, partly subjective, and purely objective. The purely subjective dimensions are perhaps the easiest; an appropriate expert estimates the position of an entity on a dimension on a 0-to-100 scale, where 0 is defined as the minimum plausible value on that dimension and 100 is defined as the maximum plausible value.

A partly subjective dimension is one in which the units of measurement are objective, but the locations of the entities must be subjectively estimated.

A wholly objective dimension is one that can be measured rather concretely, in unbiased units, before the decision. For partly or wholly objective dimensions, it is necessary to have the estimators provide not only values for each entity to be evaluated, but also minimum and maximum plausible values, in the natural units of each dimension.

The final task in Step 8 is to convert measures to the partly subjective and wholly objective dimensions, using the 0-to-100 scale in which 0 is minimum plausible and 100 is maximum plausible.

A linear transformation is almost always adequate for this purpose; errors produced by linear approximations to monotonic nonlinear functions are likely to be unimportant relative to test-retest unreliability, interrespondent differences, and the like.

It may be useful to conceptualize this step as the creation of a matrix (see Table 11-1). The importance-weighted values head each of the columns, and the programs, or action alternatives, are the rows. In Step 8 each of the cells in this

Table 11-1
Matrix: CMHC Programs of Alternatives

	A 20.1	B 11.2	C 7.9	D	E	F
Program 1						
Program 2						
Program 3						
Program 4						
Program 5						
Program 6						

matrix receives a location measure. On a subjective scale of 0 to 100 how likely is it, given what you know now, that this program (or action alternative) will maximize this value?

When all entities have been located on the relevant value dimensions, and the location measures have been rescaled; in what sense, if any, are the scales comparable? This question cannot be considered separately from the question of what "importance" means, as it was judged at Step 6. Formally, judgments at Step 6 should be designed so that when the output of Step 7 (or of Step 6, which differs only by a linear transformation) is multiplied by the output of Step 8, equal numerical distances between these products on different dimensions correspond to equal changes in desirability. For example, suppose entity A has a location of 50 and entity B a location of 10 on value dimension X, while A has a location of 70 and B a location of 90 on value dimension Y (only X and Y are relevant). Suppose further that dimension Y is twice as important as dimension X. Then, A and B should be equivalent in value. The relevant arithmetic is:

$$\text{for } A \quad 50 + 2(70) = 190$$
$$\text{for } B \quad 10 + 2(90) = 190$$

Another way of writing the same arithmetic, which makes clearer what is meant by saying that equal numerical differences between these products on different dimensions correspond to equal changes in desirability, is $(50 - 10) + 2(70 - 90) = 0$. It is important that judges understand this concept as they perform Steps 6 and 8.[1]

Step 9. Calculate utilities for entity. The equation is essentially that for a weighted average, where

$$U_i = \sum_i w_j u_{ij}$$

remembering that

$$\sum_j w_j = 100$$

U_i is the aggregate utility for the ith entity. W_j is the normalized importance weight of the jth dimension of value, and u_{ij} is the rescaled position of the ith entity on the jth dimension. Thus, w_j is the output of Step 7, and u_{ij} is the output of Step 8.

Step 10. Decide: if a single act is to be chosen, the rule is simple: maximize U_i. If a subset of i is to be chosen, then the subset for which $_i U_i$ is maximum is best.

A special case arises when one of the dimensions is subject to constraint. For example, cost may be limited by budget. In that case, Steps 4 through 10 should be done ignoring the constrained dimension. The benefit-to-cost ratios (U_i/C_i) may be calculated. Decisions should be made in decreasing order until the budget constraint is used up. (More complicated arithmetic is needed if programs are interdependent or if this rule does not come very close to exactly exhausting the budget constraint.) This is the only case in which the benefit-to-cost ratio is the appropriate figure on which to base a decision. In the absence of budget constraints, cost is just another dimension of value, to be treated on the same footing as all other dimensions of value, entering into U_i with a minus sign, like other unattractive dimensions. In general, it is the benefit-minus-cost difference, not the benefit-over-cost ratio, that should usually control decisions.

An important caveat needs to be added concerning benefit-to-cost ratios. Such ratios assume that both benefits and costs are measured on a ratio scale—a scale with a true zero point and ratio properties. The concepts, both of zero benefit and zero cost, are somewhat elusive when given close attention. An acceptable solution to the problem is to assume a value for zero-cost means, and then attempt to find the zero point on the aggregate benefit scale. If that scale is reasonably densely populated with candidate programs, an approach to locating that zero point is to ask the decisionmaker "Would you undertake this program if it had the same benefits it has now, but had zero cost?" If the answer is yes, the program is above the zero point on the benefit scale. If the answer is no, it is below the zero point.

The multiattribute utility approach can easily be adapted to cases in which there are minimum or maximum acceptable values on a given dimension of value. This can be done by simply excluding alternatives that lead to outcomes that transgress these limits.

Interpersonal and Intergroup Disagreements

There is nothing in the preceding discussions to ensure that different respondents will come up with similar numbers—and such agreements are indeed rare. Although multiattribute utility measurements can reduce the magnitude of disagreements, they cannot and should not eliminate them.

Two kinds of disagreements are distinguishable. Disagreement occurring at Steps 5 and 6 seem to be the essence of conflicting values and should be respected as much as possible. For that reason, it is advised that the judges who perform these steps should be part of the peer review process, aided by citizen participation. Considerable discussion, persuasion, and information exchange should be used in an attempt to reduce the disagreements as much as possible.

Groups can adopt various rules for decisionmaking. In the weight-averaging spirit of multiattribute utility measurement, a weight can be assigned to each of the disagreeing parties and weighted-average importance weights can be calculated.

If no rule is made to resolve disagreement, the evaluation is carried through separately for each of the disagreeing individuals or groups. Thus, the same data can lead citizen groups with different values to come to different conclusions. Then the familiar political processes, the means by which society functions in spite of conflicting interests, come into play.

Disagreements about the location of entities evaluated (Step 8) seem to be essentially like disagreements among different thermometers measuring the same temperature. If the disparity is not too great, one has little compunction about taking an average. If it is, then one is likely to suspect that some of the thermometers are not working properly. In general, the judgmentally determined location measures should reflect expertise, and typically different value dimensions should require different kinds of expertise and therefore different experts. In some practical contexts, the problem of disagreement at Step 8 can be avoided entirely by the simple expedient of asking only the best available expert for each dimension to make judgments about that dimension.

Rating and Ranking Dimensions of Values in Face-to-face Groups

Face-to-face groups, within an agency, have proven to be quite useful in generating the dimensions of values. Individuals frequently agree more about the values than they would predict. Since no values are excluded, the value dimension generation process is often useful in providing information about their own values to members of a group.

When there are groups that clearly have different values inside and outside the program which is to be evaluated, it is often useful to have each group generate its own values independently. Then, information about these values can be provided to each group. Again, it is important to emphasize that, since at this stage there is no judgment of the relative importance of the information generated, this information is useful and unthreatening to each group.

Steps 5 and 6 can be accomplished either by face-to-face groups or by individuals whose rankings are later combined. Generally, the face-to-face group process is better, if it is possible, because it tends to build a group consensus on the ordering of the values. However, when there are clearly diverse groups, within and outside a CMHC, it is most useful to permit each of these groups (or representatives of them) to perform their own rank ordering and importance weighting as a face-to-face group.

It is useful for three reasons. First, each group builds a consensus about its own values vis-à-vis the programs. This makes it possible to exchange information about the relative ordering of values between groups, so that discussions between these groups about value differences can be quite explicit and easily quantified. This pleasantly cuts down the noise of rhetoric. Second, the same evaluation data can be fed back into each group. The same data, in a matrix in which values, rank order, and/or importance weights differ considerably, will yield very different final conclusions and decisions. Thus, a number of groups can, using the same data, come to very different conclusions about whether a certain program meets their goals. This then provides them with a substantive basis for discussion with one another. Third, consensus is not a sine qua non of the evaluation process. If a number of different groups generate very different values, data must be gathered that indicate how contemplated actions bear on every one of the values. This forces the evaluation researcher into multiple measurement. In addition, it means that decisionmakers receive research data on issues that may be foreign to their own values, but quite germane to the values of other groups, i.e., persons affected by a program. The result of this value diversity is a much greater richness of evaluation information from which concerned groups benefit.

At Step 8, the best choice is to use experts to determine the measurement of the entity being evaluated on each dimension. At the planning stage one presumes that whatever research or other evaluation data are available must be combined in some way to generate a location measure. Therefore, it is best to use individuals who are able to make such judgments expertly.

The Integration of Planning and Evaluation

Earlier, it was asserted that the planning and evaluation process could and should be integrated. How, then, does one proceed from a decision-theoretic research plan of this kind to the evaluation process?

As has been earlier noted, a matrix has been generated as part of the multiattribute utility planning process. All the values that have been rank-ordered and importance-weighted are in the matrix. The rows of the matrix consist of the programs, subprograms, etc.—i.e., the entities that are being evaluated. The columns are the value dimensions. In each cell of the matrix, there is a location judgment of the extent to which program 1 is likely to contribute to value A, etc. In the planning stage, this judgment has been made using all the data available on the program. Where programs do not exist, and potential new options are noted, these judgments are no more than educated guesses.

As the program proceeds, data are gathered. In cases in which the educated guess used in planning was specific enough to be modified by an observed number (i.e., number of participants in a voluntary program), the standard techniques of Bayesian statistics can be used to update initial guesses as data accumulate. In some cases, the value dimensions used may be so abstract that numbers observable during a program are unlikely to represent them, though they obviously have some bearing on them. In such cases, the entries in the matrix should still be updated, either by the direct use of expert judgment or by some more formal process, such as further decomposition of each value via the value hierarchy concept.

Thus, the original evaluation structure used in planning the program can also be used to evaluate it as it proceeds and to assess its merits when it is over.

However, values (here interpreted as importance weights) change as programs proceed, as circumstances change, and as time passes. The weights that are appropriate this year may not be appropriate next year. This suggests that certain evaluative questions, based on the same updated location measures, can and should be asked: How does the present program measure up to the expectations we had for it when we planned it? Given this year's values, how does the present program look? Should it be changed? If so, how?

A Device for Bringing Bayesian Tools to Bear on Evaluation Updating

It is often reasonable to define a value dimension as a goal. A very abstract dimension can often be operationalized by specifying some measure or set of measures, such that attainment of them constitutes success, and failure to attain them constitutes failure. Thus, the probability of success can be treated as the location measure and can be updated as data accumulate by standard Bayesian procedures. This technique will be illustrated in two examples, one hypothetical and one real.

A Simple Hypothesis Integrating Planning and Evaluation

A large city has a program for identifying and treating health problems, and different "models" are being evaluated. Accordingly, 400 children are randomly assigned as "clients." Staffing patterns vary among the first three models. Model 1 is staffed by one full-time medical doctor and one full-time paraprofessional; Model 2 is staffed by one half-time medical doctor and five full-time paraprofessionals; Model 3 is staffed by one doctor who works quarter-time and seven full-time paraprofessionals. Model 4 is a control, or notreatment group, and it indicates how well children do outside of the program models. Staff members are randomly assigned to the different models (except Model 4), and the models are comparable in terms of total funding level, total salaries, equipment, medicine, access to ancillary services, etc. All the children are tested on the first day of the program and retested after one year. Steps in a decision-theoretic approach to evaluation would proceed as follows. (The numbering does not correspond to that in the list of ten steps to evaluation via multiattribute utility stated earlier.)

Step 1. Identify program goals. Typically, program goals are consistent with the decisionmaker's values, and it is possible to make explicit the program's goals and their relative importance to the decisionmaker. The program has three separate goals: to improve physical health, mental health, and social competency. In many instances, such broad goals must be subdivided and partitioned into subgoals that can be assessed separately. But, this example is simplified by the assumption that these goals can be used without further elaboration. (This corresponds to Step 5 of our original list.)

Step 2. Determine the relative importance of goals. Since the hypothetical program is targeted on health problems, it is plausible to assume that improving physical health is the more important goal and social competency is the least important goal. Following our procedure, an arbitrary importance weight of 10 is assigned to the least important goal (social competency), and the remaining goals are weighed relative to the least important goal. It is assumed that the relative importance of these goals is expressed by weights of 10 (social competency), 20 (mental health), and 80 (physical health). (This corresponds to Step 6 of our original list.)

Step 3. Identify probabilistic measures of goal attainment. In this step, operational definitions of the program's goals are specified. The appropriate measures may be very complex and difficult to measure, or they may be simply defined and amenable to measurement. For this example simple, dichotomous goals are used, and the criterion for success will be whether a client exceeds predefined standards. For each goal, the location measure will be the probability that a (randomly chosen) client will exceed the standard.

Step 4. Estimate prior probabilities of goal attainment. Prior to implementation of programs, there are typically few or no data about program maximization of goals. Nevertheless, decisionmakers have subjective prior probabilities that should guide the planning process and govern the selection of activities. Guttentag (1973) refers to a planning process built on wholly subjective, prior information. For the present example, the subjective prior probabilities for each goal are given in Table 11-2. These prior probabilities suggest an initial

Table 11-2
Subjective Prior Probabilities for Each Goal

| Model | Prior Probability of Client Achieving Goal | | | Prior Utility |
	Goal 1	Goal 2	Goal 3	
Model 1	0.40	0.80	0.60	54.00
Model 2	0.40	0.75	0.50	52.00
Model 3	0.30	0.60	0.45	40.50
Model 4	0.10	0.30	0.35	17.50

expectation that Model 1 is the best according to all goals, except that it is equal in value to Model 2 in terms of achieving the physical health goal. (This corresponds to Step 8 of our original list.)

Step 5. Calculate prior utilities. In this example, the worth of a model will be determined by (1) the expected number of clients who achieve each goal, and (2) the importance of each goal. Since the expected number is proportional to the prior probability, the prior utility for each model is:

$$U_i = \sum_j (W_j \cdot P_{ij})$$

where W_j is the weight for the *j*th goal, and P_{ij} is the prior probability that a client in the *i*th model will achieve the *j*th goal. The prior utility for a given model is proportional to the sum of the prior probabilities, with each multiplied by the appropriate importance weight.

Step 6. Measure goal attainment. In this example, there is an operational definition of goals, and pertinent data are frequency counts of goal achievement on retest. For the hypothetical example, it is assumed that the proportions are given in Table 11-3. Clearly, these data run counter to prior expectations on goals 2 and 3. Models 2 and 3 do better than Model 1. The computation, in Step 8, of posterior utilities will indicate how these data should change prior opinion about the value of these models.

Step 7. Calculate posterior probabilities. Before posterior utilities can be calculated, it is appropriate to revise the probabilities associated with goal attainment. Bayes' theorem (Edwards, Lindman, and Savage 1963) is the algorithm used to revise probabilities; the beta distribution is used as a prior distribution in this example. Since the assessment of prior distributions can be controversial, it is arbitrarily assumed that the parameters of the prior Beta distribution sum to 1.0. (This amounts to assuming that all prior opinions were very weakly held.) Using the prior distribution and the probabilities of the data for each model (described by the binomial distribution), the posterior probabilities (means of the posterior distributions) shown in Table 11-4 are derived. (Note that the posterior probabilities in Table 11-5 are very nearly equal to the

Table 11-3
Proportion of Clients Achieving Goal

| Model | Proportion of Clients Achieving Goal | | |
	Goal 1	Goal 2	Goal 3
Model 1	62/100	40/100	40/100
Model 2	55/100	85/100	50/100
Model 3	35/100	90/100	65/100
Model 4	10/100	35/100	40/100

Table 11-4
Posterior Probabilities of Client Achieving Goal

Model	Posterior Probabilities of Client Achieving Goal			Posterior Utility
	Goal 1	Goal 2	Goal 3	
Model 1	0.62	0.41	0.41	61.90
Model 2	0.55	0.86	0.51	66.30
Model 3	0.35	0.91	0.66	52.80
Model 4	0.10	0.35	0.40	19.00

sample proportions in Table 11-4. This is an example of "stable estimation," since data exert a much larger effect on the posteriors than the priors do. If, however, there is little or no sample information, the posterior probabilities will be close to the prior probabilities. Thus, this method reflects the diagnosticity of data from program evaluation, and provides a mathematically appropriate rule for modifying opinion about programs.)

Step 8. Calculate posterior utilities. The computational formula for posterior utilities is (except for minor notational changes) identical to the equation in Step 6 for calculating posterior utilities. Replace the prior probabilities in Step 5 with the posterior probabilities from Step 7. The posterior utilities are shown in Table 11-4.

This hypothetical example illustrates (1) how evaluation data can be directly related to the decisionmaker's values, and (2) how these data can be used to revise prior assessments of the worth of the programs. By assessing the worth of each model across all dimensions, the utility score incorporates trade-offs between goals or values. Note, for example, that Model 2 has a higher overall posterior utility than Model 1, although Model 1 has a somewhat higher posterior probability on Goal 1 than Model 2 does. These data indicate that the data from evaluation should induce the decisionmaker to rate Model 2 as a better investment than Model 1, and reverse the prior rank ordering.

An Example from the Career Education Project

Currently, a decision-theoretic approach is being used by a career education project (ETR). A goal of this project is to reach potential members of the labor force, especially "home-based" women, and counsel them about career education or training opportunities. One way of evaluating this project is to specify goals in terms of status in education or training activities. The general approach can be illustrated using data from a formative stage of the project; e.g., follow-up for clients who terminated the service with the stated intention of enrolling in an education or training activity. (The tentative plans are for the latest evaluation to include a control group and a more complete set of goals.) For the follow-up study, the goals and importance weights (in parentheses) are: Goal 1, client enrolled and completed ETR (90); Goal 2, client enrolled and participating in ETR (60); Goal 3, client enrolled and waiting for ETR to begin (30); Goal 4, client tried to enroll but failed to resolve constraints (15); and Goal 5, client enrolled but dropped ETR (10).

To evaluate the differential impact of the counseling service on different subgroups of clients, many comparative analyses were made. Utility is calculated for each separate subgroup. For example, high school graduates were compared to nongraduates. After appropriate instructions, subjective prior probability estimates were determined by a project member. These, along with the prior utilities (calculated from Step 5), are shown in Table 11-5.

These prior probabilities were subjective estimates of what goal attainment would be six months after clients left the service. Data for these clients were obtained by talking with them after the leave of six months. Actual results are indicated in 11-6, which shows the posterior probabilities and utilities.

Murphy (1974) has suggested that comparing prior and posterior probabilities may highlight ways in which the program is not performing as expected. Disparity between the wholly subjective priors and the data-based posteriors could indicate that the program should be modified, or that additional research efforts might be required. In particular, such analyses may show that a program should be modified to better meet the needs of specific subgroups of clients.

Table 11-5
Prior Probabilities of Client Achieving Goal

Comparison Group	Prior Probability of Client Achieving Goal					Prior Utility
	Goal 1	Goal 2	Goal 3	Goal 4	Goal 5	
Graduates	0.23	0.30	0.10	0.07	0.30	45.75
Nongraduates	0.15	0.22	0.06	0.12	0.45	34.80

Table 11-6
Posterior Probabilities of Client Achieving Goal

Comparison Group	Posterior Probability of Client Achieving Goal					Posterior Utility
	Goal 1	Goal 2	Goal 3	Goal 4	Goal 5	
Graduates	0.21	0.45	0.05	0.11	0.18	50.85
Nongraduates	0.29	0.30	0.01	0.19	0.21	49.35

In these analyses of the follow-up studies, no control group or randomization was used. Thus, self-selection among clients is a distinct possibility. Nevertheless, utility measures such as these indicate how classes of clients are interacting with the program and—regardless of their personal or demographic characteristics—indicate differences in outcomes for client groups. Thus, the utility scores are useful, even under nonexperimental conditions.

These illustrations show how the method discussed in this chapter can be used in both nonexperimental and experimental conditions. This flexibility is a major advantage over more conventional approaches, which are generally unrelated to planning or resource allocation decisions.

An evaluation paradigm has been presented that makes it formally possible to use citizen participation and the peer review process as an integral part of CMHC evaluations. This paradigm incorporates multiple measurement, data inclusiveness, continuous feedback, and the potential integration of catchment demography with measures of program effectiveness.

Note

1. Personal communication from Mr. Howard Davis.

References

Edwards, W., 1971. "Social Utilities," in *The Engineering Economist*, Summer Symposium Series. 6.

_____ ; Guttentag, M.; and Snapper, K. 1975. "A Decision-theoretic Approach to Evaluation Research," in *Handbook of Evaluation Research*, edited by E. Struening and M. Guttentag, vol. 1, Beverly Hills, Calif.: Sage Publications.

_____ ; Lindman, H.; and Savage, L.J. 1963. "Bayesian Statistical Inference for Psychological Research." *Psychological Review* 70:193-242.

Guttentag, M. 1973. "Subjectivity and Its Use in Evaluation Research." *Evaluation* 1(2).

Murphy, J.F. 1974. "Multi-Attribute Utility Analysis: An Application in Social Utilities." *Career Education Project Technical Report 74-1.*

12 Evaluation—An Ethical Perspective

David Allen

The preceding chapters in Part II have described some of the methodological and technical aspects of evaluation as applied to mental health services. However, evaluation is a rational exercise which always takes place in a strongly political context. It is used to provide data to facilitate the decisionmaking process at all levels of bureaucracy and includes legislators, administrators, and consumers. Weiss (1973) emphasizes this when she states, "... evaluation deals with programs which are the creation of political decisions. These programs were proposed, defined, debated, enacted and funded through political processes, and in implementation they remain subject to pressures, both supportive and hostile, that arise out of the play of politics."

The harsh reality is that mental health evaluation can exert a powerful influence on decisions relating to the funding of new services or the elimination of existing programs. It may have a devastating effect on the availability of mental health services for all consumers, but especially on needy persons without a strong political base. On the other hand, effective evaluation within a good organizational structure can directly influence the standard of care by stimulating administrators and staff to correct the deficiencies outlined by the evaluation.

Thus, evaluation is a powerful tool which has the potential for improving the availability and quality of mental health care. But it may be abused by being used to satisfy personal biases or prejudices against certain groups of people and special programs. Therefore, the evaluator, whether involved in management information, monitoring, research, or clinical inspection, has a grave responsibility to ensure that one's work is not only technically competent but is conducted with the highest standard of professional ethics.

How then can this ethical perspective be introduced and maintained in mental health evaluation?

From the viewpoint of a clinical inspector, I suggest that in examining his/her ethical responsibility, the evaluator should consider at least five major areas: the facts, quasi-theological basis, moral reasoning, loyalties, and implementation.

The Facts

The evaluator must be committed to seeking the facts at all costs. For it is the collection of accurate data and the honest interpretation of these salient facts which provide competent evaluation and good ethics.

131

The ideal evaluator may be compared to Firth's ideal observer. According to Firth (1952), the ideal observer should be omniscient, omnipercipient, disinterested, dispassionate, consistent, and otherwise normal.

In striving toward omniscience, the evaluator must aim to be technically competent and involved in an ongoing educational process. He/she should be committed to gather the facts from all available sources including previous evaluation reports, management information systems, clinical inspection and research based on naturalistic and experimental designs. The work should be comprehensive in scope, addressing as many aspects of the program as possible. This may include administration and management, physical facilities, accessibility and visibility, staff qualifications and function, patient care, direct services, treatment modalities, record keeping, continuity of care, consultation and education, coordination with other agencies, etc.

The evaluator should be familiar with not only the facts from his/her own field but also those related to the multidisciplinary influences upon his/her work. This may involve consultation from experts skilled in the social, cultural, ethical, and political parameters of the evaluation process.

To approach omnipercipience the evaluator should try to understand how the program being evaluated is perceived by and affects all the different parties involved. For example, how can a program be evaluated without obtaining the patients' view of the care received? Traditionally, however, the staff or director's perspective has predominated in the evaluation of mental health services. In a descriptive study by the author of mental health centers in Massachusetts, a patient advocate (mental health paraprofessional) sampled consumers' opinions about the mental health services in their respective catchment areas, with questions such as "Where would you take a relative who had a case of nerves?" or "What are the mental health services in your catchment area?" It was surprising to find that, in the majority of cases, few people knew about the mental health services in their community. In one outstanding example, a police officer in a small town did not know where the day hospital was located, even though it was right above the police station. This indicates a failure of the program to be accessible to its potential consumer and underscores the need for consultation with the police to enhance program outreach and effectiveness.

Therefore, evaluation must involve input from staff, patients, families, consumers on the street, charity groups, churches, etc., in order to present a true picture of the quality, accessibility, and extent of services in the program.

The evaluator, like the ideal observer, should seek to be disinterestedly interested and dispassionately passionate. This means the withdrawal of particular interests and passions so that one can be interested in and passionate to the whole. Such objectivity is almost impossible, especially if the evaluator is paid by the same agency that is being evaluated. For example a conflict of interests is often experienced by evaluators hired by the state to assess its own programs. However, a relative state of disinterestedness and dispassionateness could be achieved by using a team approach to evaluation. The team should consist of clinicians, social scientists, consumers, ex-patients, and other interested persons. Thus, the interplay of the different interests and passions of the members of the team will tend to reduce the possibility of particular interests or passions controlling the evaluation process. This particular team method was most successful in our evaluation of a large state hospital in Massachusetts. The evaluation process, involving professionals, citizens, staff, and legislators, even after the evaluation was completed, produced a united constituency which continues to fight for needed reform in the hospital.

However, the multidisciplinary approach is not without conflict because of the different backgrounds and levels of training of the participants. The professional evaluator in the group must seek to educate the other members of the team in the basic principles of the evaluation and outline whatever standards are available. One should seek to create a feeling of closeness and open expression in the group. The group should then establish common goals, e.g., normalization of the patient. Only after such preparation should the evaluation begin. This process demands decisiveness, understanding, and tolerance on the part of the professional evaluator. Nevertheless, multidisciplinary evaluation is a powerful educational and consciousness-raising process, which can function as a most effective agent of change. No doubt this will become a greater trend in light of the demand for more public accountability and citizen participation.

The demands of evaluation are such that the evaluator should demonstrate a sense of consistency in all aspects of the process. He/she should be consistent in the planning, preparation, procedure, and presentation of the work. This does not involve a rigid, inflexible attitude; but it implies a sincere commitment to the fair treatment of all involved individuals. The evaluator should be dependable and persistent in maintaining high standards of performance in all situations. This is sometimes very difficult because of close relationships, personal biases, the subjective nature of the evaluation process, and conflicts of interests. For example, state evaluators are expected to be harder on the private institutions which they license than on the often antiquated, inefficient human warehouses that the state maintains. This is a double standard which places the evaluator in an awkward situation.

The final characteristic of the ideal observer is that he/she should be otherwise normal. In essence this means that he/she is a "normal person," the implication being that the evaluator is an individual with limited knowledge, expertise, and ability to act. Thus, he/she is subject periodically to failure through ignorance, incompetence, and misinterpretation of data. But, it is failure that may also serve to underscore the evaluator's responsibility to recognize one's limitations and to allow the work to be examined in an atmosphere of openness and consultation with others. As Elaine Cumming said, the best check on our work is to let it be examined by our nicest enemy.

Quasi-theological Basis

Evaluation must involve more than the collection of factual data. The facts must be related to the human ethical perspective in order to serve the best interests of the individual.

"Values always accompany and give special psychological significance to facts and when we deprive facts of their value, we fabricate artifacts which have no reality in human psychology. An individual may suspend his value judgment when he wants to examine a fact from a specific point of view, but then the ethical content has to be reestablished if the fact is to have human significance. If we remove the ethical dimension we reduce man to a subhuman animal . . ." (Arieti 1975).

Therefore, the evaluator must be cognizant of his/her personal ethical value system and its relation to those being served. What one believes about the nature of people exerts a subtle but controlling influence on attitudes, behavior, and treatment of individuals. According to Eisenberg (1972), "What we believe of men affects the behavior of men for it determines what each expects from each other. Theories of education, of political science, and economics and the very politics of government are based on implied concepts of man."

For example, the evaluator cannot apply the principle of reciprocity (the Golden Rule) if he/she believes that other people should not be treated with the same dignity and respect that he himself expects. During an evaluation of a community mental health center by our team, a mental health administrator said, "Even though the state hospital environment is substandard, it is suitable for chronic mentally ill patients because they don't need anything better." His value system must affect his attitude toward the treatment of chronic patients and hence his commitment to reform in mental health.

For the most part, Western ethics are based on the Judeo-Christian tradition which at its heart claims that human beings are created in the image of God. This *imago dei* is the basis for personhood, dignity, and human rights. It is this quality of inestimable value in individuals which enhances personal meaning, interpersonal relationships, and human community.

All individuals, regardless of mental illness or other disabilities, must be seen as persons first, deserving the utmost respect and concern. For example, the individual with schizophrenia should be seen not merely as a 'schizophrenic' but as a person who has problems in mental functioning. And so we, too, are persons who have problems in other areas of life. Therefore, our relationship with the mentally ill must be based on the acceptance of our common personhood— rather than on our diverse problems. This is the meaning of Buber's I-thou relationship as opposed to the dehumanized I-it or subject-object interaction. Thus, the Judeo-Christian ethic, above all, demands that we see in each other the person, that is, the shared human qualities inherent in us all. This makes the Golden Rule a practical reality, i.e., doing unto others as you would have them do unto you.

However, the moral responsibility inherent in this reciprocal, empathic relationship among persons requires allegiance to other vital principles, such as trust, forgiveness, truth telling, love, promise keeping, justice, liberty and noninjury. These principles are so germane to the human community that they may be called the "constitutive imperatives," i.e., principles upon which all laws governing society are made. Jonsen and Butler (1975) emphasize the importance of this concept:

Respect for individuals requires that every individual be treated in consideration of his uniqueness, equal to every other, and that special justification is required for interference with their purposes, their privacy or their behavior. It implies sets of liberties, rights and duties, and obligations especially of promise-keeping and truth-telling.

The evaluator, in order to be true to the human ethical perspective in his/her work, must continually place himself/herself in the position of the client—feeling what the client feels and then treating him as the evaluator would personally like to be treated. The ethical dynamic is that if the services are not of the quality acceptable to the evaluator or his/her family, then they are not appropriate for the client. As a result, the moral imperative is that the evaluator should be committed to a process of constructive change to make the services available to the patient personally acceptable.

Moral Reasoning

The moral reasoning involved in evaluation, or any other process, has a profound influence on the way persons are treated. Therefore, the evaluator is obligated to be aware of and to constantly examine the types of moral reasoning operating in his/her work.

There are many different forms of moral reasoning, ranging from the less complex mode of ethical egoism in Kohlberg's stage 1 to the more sophisticated mode of formalism of universal ethical principle in stage 6. The author has found it particularly helpful to examine the moral reasoning involved in his work in light of Kohlberg's (1973) stages of moral development. However, the evaluator has to confront two major conflicting forms of moral reasoning: utilitarianism and the equal-value view of life.

Although there are many varieties of utilitarianism, its essence can be summed up as "the greatest good for the greatest number." Though it is appealing, it offers nothing for those who are not a part of the greatest number. This may help explain the atrocities inflicted by biomedical technology on certain minorities—the mentally ill, the mentally retarded and the racially outcast. The inhumane treatment of institutionalized mentally ill persons, the unethical Tuskegee syphilitic study performed on unknowing black men, the injection of potentially lethal hepatitis virus into mentally retarded persons at

Willowbrook State Hospital in New York, and the negligent care of the elderly in many state facilities and nursing homes are but a few examples of the treatment shown to those minorities who are assumed to be expendable for the greatest good. This mode of moral reasoning is particularly attractive in times of fiscal crisis during an economic depression. As a result, in state budget debates, human-service components are more vulnerable to being cut than public works or transportation programs.

The greatest-good-for-the-greatest-number concept has the inherent assumption that only life of a certain quality is worthwhile. Thus, there is a tendency to define personhood on the basis of whether utility outweighs disutility. And whenever the utility/disutility balance is upset, one's worth as a person decreases. For example, becoming mentally ill reduces utility; as a result, the person becomes subject to a barrage of indignities and loss of human rights, manifested by dehumanizing conditions, lack of treatment, inadequate rehabilitation, and job discrimination.

This is contradictory to the human ethical perspective; under the euphemism of the public good, it implies a merit view of justice, denying positive presumption, due process, and equality. This strains the moral fiber of the society itself and undermines the meaning of those indispensable humanizing qualities of love, compassion, justice, and liberty for its members. Eventually this leads to a society, or better still a "nonsociety," which is insensitive to its weak. Thus, only the powerful are strong, and they are strong only as long as they have power, e.g., Nazi Germany.

In contrast the equal-value view of life assumes that all individuals, regardless of their utility/disutility ratio, are persons who have an equal claim to dignity, respect, and human rights. Thus, all persons have utility—but utility must never define personhood and the right to life, liberty, and good in the world. The emotionally ill, the racial minority, mentally retarded, and the elderly are persons deserving equal treatment regardless of their power base in society. Justice demands an equal consideration of each person's claim, regardless of the person or the situation. This demands that the powerful in society share their power base with those who have none, making advantages for even the most disadvantaged.

As the movement for public accountability and governmental regulation of services continues to gather momentum, the evaluator will be in even greater demand. But this increased demand or status is concomitant with an even greater responsibility to the public good. As a result, the evaluator will be pressured to use his/her expertise to satisfy the whims and fancies of those in power rather than to represent the interest of those in need. It seems so easy to adapt to a utilitarian philosophy of the greatest good for the greatest number—or the most powerful. Yet, in reality, we do well to remember that the mentally ill, the disabled, are an integral part of human society. They are a part of us, and we are a part of them. The way we treat them is a direct reflection of the humanity and quality of life we espouse, for their destiny is inextricably linked to our own. Therefore, the evaluator of services for mentally ill persons, who have suffered so ignominously, must be a guardian of the human ethical dynamic in society. This can only be done effectively if the moral reasoning involved in his/her work leads to the enhancement of the dignity of all persons—especially those in need.

Loyalties

Our loyalties dictate the ultimate ends we serve in our work. "For where your treasure is, there will your heart be also." Therefore, the evaluator must face the question: To whom and to what am I responsible? One must examine where his/her basic loyalties lie in relationship to his/her means and ends.

Ethically speaking, the true purpose of life is that all individuals, including the mentally ill, may experience the meaning and fulfillment of their personhood, dignity, and human rights. This demands a strong commitment because all else in life must function as a means to that end.

Quality mental health care is more an entity to be desired than defined. However, it does imply a form of service or treatment which enhances the dignity and respect of the individual for one's own person and the personhood of others, so that he/she is able to function to the fullest in the community. Obviously, not only does this involve helping the individual to appreciate his/her own worth, autonomy, and responsibilities, but it also simultaneously demands a commitment to a change process to institute more ideal justice structures in the surrounding society. This is the quintessence of community mental health in its ideal form. Therefore, mental health evaluation, like administration and direct care, should be seen as a means to enhance the quality of mental health care for all individuals so that they may experience the meaning and fulfillment of their personhood, dignity, and human rights.

This perspective is of the utmost importance. Whenever a means, even with the best intentions, becomes an end in itself, persons are dehumanized, even destroyed. Thus, whenever the evaluation process becomes an end in itself, a vicious cycle is set up and the human ethical perspective is lost. Thus, it behooves the responsible evaluator to constantly examine his/her motivation and loyalties in all aspects of the work process. This may mean refusing to perform certain types of evaluation or exercising caution in widespread distribution of certain data. For example, a well-known mental health evaluator who shall be nameless was enraged when he discovered that a certain government agency intended to use the results of his evaluation to withdraw funding from a particular program. He said that his intention was the improvement rather than the reduction of services. Many direct-care providers claim that they are finding it more difficult to devote the desired time to patient care because of the increased pressure of paper work to comply with the demand for evaluation and regulation. I have found evidence of this in my experience with evaluating community mental health centers. The fact is that if evaluation interrupts the delivery of clinical care, it has become an end in itself, and the patient is being cheated. This is blatantly unethical because we may end up with good data but shoddy patient care. Therefore, in order to prevent this catastrophe, we must reach a healthy balance between good evaluative techniques and the delivery of optimum patient care. As an evaluator, I find the admonition of Howard Davis at the First New England Conference on Evaluation to be very helpful—K.I.S.S.: Keep it simple, stupid.

Implementation

In the area of implementation, "where the action is," the evaluator must tread cautiously with wisdom, understanding, and openness to new information, and methods.

Before implementation, the evaluator should ask himself/herself questions, such as, "What is my basic motivation for carrying out this evaluation? How will the data be used? Will the evaluation enhance the human dignity of the persons involved? Would I object to the procedure being applied to myself, my family, or others close to me? Do I have proper informed consent from the persons involved? Can I universalize my actions (i.e., what would happen if everyone acted as I do?)?

From an ethical perspective action and motivation are inseparable. The requirement for both is justice, mercy, and humility. Micah, the Hebrew prophet, describes it well: "What, O Man, does the Lord require of Thee but to do justice, love mercy and walk humbly with God" (Old Testament, Micah 6:8). This provides an excellent guide to the evaluator when considering the implementation of technique. He/she must act justly. This involves treating all persons fairly with the highest standards of technical excellence. He/she should be convinced that the evaluation is a genuine effort to gather data as a means to improve care rather than a bureaucratic defense against facing the problem and instituting the appropriate action or reform. For example, where only one staff member is appointed to care for forty severely retarded persons (found wallowing in urine), there is no need for further study or evaluation of the quality of their care. The only ethically acceptable response in this situation is action, i.e., more funds, more staff, or better environment.

The evaluator must be merciful and compassionate, treating others as he/she would want to be treated, sharing his power base with those who have none. However, compassion demands action beyond the technique and process of evaluation. It requires commitment to correct the deficiencies pointed out by the evaluation. Far too often, evaluation reports become dusty ornaments on the shelves of administrators. The evaluator whose ongoing concern is assurance of quality care has a responsibility that ends only when action is taken to correct the deficiencies outlined by his/her work.

Because the dilemmas are many, knowledge limited and solutions few, the evaluator has ample cause to be humble. Many variables which cannot be evaluated effectively, e.g., trust, caring, understanding, etc., are nonetheless important factors in human relationships. There are no absolute measures for evaluating the quality of mental health services. The evaluator cannot hope to be totally scientific, but can only aim to apply systematic and quantitative techniques to measure standards which are so often based on unproved assumptions and opinions. For what may be considered good today may be found not to be in the best interest of the patient tomorrow. Considering then the inconclusive nature of evaluation in the ever-changing field of mental health, the evaluator must always be willing to seek consultation from higher and better authority. He/she should be searching for new ideas and better techniques to improve skills, in order to enhance the development of better services for all persons.

As evaluators, whether concerned with monitoring, research, or clinical inspection, we do well to heed the warning of Donald T. Campbell, President-elect of the American Psychological Association (Campbell, 1973):

Many of the things that we know are good and should be done will not occur in natural laboratories where we will be able to evaluate them. So let us be focused on action, let us be focused on making changes. Where possible, we would like to know what the effects of these changes are. But we mustn't allow this to be a sabotage of action, like setting up a committee to study it."

In conclusion, the evaluator has both a sacred responsibility and a moral obligation to be constantly aware of the ethical perspective of his/her work. He or she must be committed to the highest standard of ethical practice so that the evaluation process becomes a humanizing force to liberate the mentally ill person, who has suffered too long under the oppressive and dehumanizing forces of society.

References

Arieti, S. 1975. "Psychiatric Controversy: Man's Ethical Dimension." *American Journal of Psychiatry* 132:1.

Campbell, D. 1973. "Experimentation Revisited—Interview with Susan Salasin." *Evaluation* 1:7.

Cumming, E. 1976. "Some Problems Encountered in Attempts to Evaluate Mental Health Programs," in *Trends in Mental Health Evaluation*, Edited by E. Markson and D. Allen. Lexington, Mass.: Lexington Books.

Eisenberg, L. 1972. "The Human Nature of Human Nature." *Science* Vol 176. No. 4031.

Firth, R. 1952. "Ethical Absolutism and the Ideal Observer." *Philosophy and Phenomenological Research* 12:317-345.

Jonsen, A., and Butler, L. 1975. "Public Ethics and Policy Making." *Hastings Center Report* 5:25.

Kohlberg, L. 1973. "The Claim to Moral Adequacy of a Highest Stage of Moral Development." *Journal of Philosophy* 30:630-646.

Weiss, C. 1973. "Where Politics and Evaluation Research Meet." *Evaluation* 1:37.

Appendix:
Self-Corrective Feedback
through Evaluation—
Some New England
Examples

In May 1975, the New England Conference on Evaluation and Mental Health Services was held in Boston, Massachusetts. An integral part of the conference included descriptions of evaluation programs currently underway in a variety of settings. This appendix provides a brief overview of some ongoing work in New England—in both the public sector and the private sectors. Obviously, this is not an all-inclusive overview of evaluation research and management information systems in use in the Northeast. Rather, salient features of the evaluative efforts at the state level are summarized for two states and for two private, nonprofit psychiatric hospitals. The description of ongoing mental health evaluations in Maine provides a useful example of a relevant system—developed at the local level of the community mental health center—that is potentially useful statewide. New Hampshire's program focuses on (1) development of that necessary, but not sufficient, tool for program evaluation, the management information system, (2) management by objectives, and (3) PSRO (Professional Standards Review Organization). Butler and McLean have developed somewhat more sophisticated evaluation research programs, perhaps because private nonprofit psychiatric hospitals have had a history of greater commitment to and support of such work than has traditionally existed in the public sector. Each system differs from the others in staffing, focus of effort, base populations served, and available resources for evaluation. Yet all share a concern with some form of self-corrective feedback through evaluation—whether at the facility or state level.

Maine

The Maine Mental Health Information System Project, supported in part by funds from the National Institute of Mental Health (NIMH), is intended to develop a comprehensive information system which would provide data both for management purposes and for evaluation.

This system is being developed in a series of successive components. The first component is to provide management information, i.e. information to be used for decisionmaking concerning individual employees, individual clients, or local management policies. The initial emphasis of the management information system is on fiscal accountability: to provide for billing, accounts receivable, accounting, unit costing, and other functions necessary to understanding the

Edited from papers presented by Charles W. Acker, David E. Askew, Mollie C. Grob, Stuart P. Howell, and Richard Longabaugh.

operation and ensuring its economic survival. A second aspect of the management information system is staff-activity accounting—to provide data on how staff spend their time. The third aspect is that of client statistics, providing information on demographic characteristics of clients, the problems they present, the services they receive, and information as to changes that take place during the course of treatment.

Since the management information system module has gotten underway, more focus has been placed on development of the evaluation module (which includes baseline data, performance statistics, and measures of client change to assess outcome). The following will be a review of the development of the outcome evaluation component of the Community Mental Health Center (CMHC) in Aroostook, Maine. Designed as a two-year project, its purpose was to develop and pilot a total management-information and outcome-evaluation system at Aroostook that could be used by Community Mental Health Centers and state mental health facilities on a statewide basis.

The first issue addressed in development of the outcome evaluation component of the total project was selection of a method for gathering information regarding the impact of mental health services on people receiving them. It became apparent almost immediately that, given the resources and the time available, development of an original instrument for measurement of treatment outcome was out of the question. Consequently, two existing techniques were selected: (1) Goal Attainment Scaling, and (2) the Denver Community Mental Health Outcome Questionnaire. Factors considered in deciding on these two instruments included: (1) the demonstrated validity and reliability of the two instruments; (2) the generic nature of the two instruments; (3) the meaningfulness of the data contained in the two instruments to treatment staff; and (4) the potential adaptability of the two instruments for use as clinician report or self-report instruments.

The Maine Management Information System was an attempt to design a system that could be used statewide. This required that it be both efficient and inexpensive. Thus, it was decided to attempt to incorporate Goal Attainment Scaling into treatment records, thereby eliminating the need for one set of records to document the progress of treatment and a separate set to measure treatment outcome. The format for treatment recording has been set up so that after general treatment information—including the presenting problem, the circumstances of the referral, a selection of proposed treatment modalities, long-range goals, and proposed coordination with other treatment services—a set of problem areas are identified. A separate page in the record is then set aside for each problem area. The problem is specifically defined, goals related to the problem are scaled according to Goal Attainment scaling norms, a treatment plan for the specific problem is indicated, and progress toward the goals is noted contact by contact.

The treatment record as described above is reviewed after the third contact with the patient, ninety days after intake, and every ninety days after that. At each ninety-day review, treatment goals and treatment plans are revised as necessary. It is hoped that systematic and frequent reviews will counterbalance inevitable bias—stemming from the fact that treatment staff are setting and evaluating goals for their own clients. It is also planned that third party interviewer follow-ups will be conducted on randomly selected records, and the results of these interviews will be compared with the progress towards goals noted by treatment staff. It is hoped that this will serve as another balance against the possibility of biased reporting, which might occur were treatment staff to set goals and evaluate patient progress themselves.

Future plans revolve around the use of the data generated by the Goal Attainment Record Keeping System and the beginning of implementation of the Denver Community Mental Health Outcome Questionnaire. At the present time, it is planned that, at the time a case is terminated, the patient's initial and final level of goal attainment in each problem area will be entered into the master file of the Management Information System. This will allow initial levels of goal attainment, final levels of goal attainment, and change scores to be computed across clients, across programs, and by individual treatment staff. Future plans also include the coding of problems so that change scores can be computed across problem areas and across treatment modalities. Entering the goal attainment scores into the master record for each client would allow for many other kinds of comparisons to be made. Goal attainment scores may be compared for different age groups, different levels of education, different levels of income, etc. Such comparisons would be made on a selective basis in an attempt to address specific questions regarding differential responsiveness to mental health services.

New Hampshire

The Division of Mental Health is one of three divisions in the State Department of Health and Welfare; the other two are the Division of Welfare and the Division of Public Health. Within the Division of Mental Health, the Office of Community Mental Health has responsibility for the development and operation of services for the mentally ill and emotionally disturbed. Neither the Central Office nor any of the components of the Division of Mental Health—with the exception of the Office of Community Mental Health—has efforts underway to establish methods of service evaluation.

The Division of Mental Health has found that it can no longer account for the expenditure of state dollars by merely reciting the numbers of people who are "seen," numbers of interviews conducted, etc. The State Legislature, to whom it is accountable, wants to know how the money is spent, and more importantly, what effect the expenditures have had on the mental health problems toward which the services have been directed.

Accordingly, the first part of New Hampshire's statewide mental health program evaluation system is a Management Information System relating to patient admission and termination information. Although there has been a statewide community mental health statistical data system for the past ten years, it has only been in the past year or two that it has been used for evaluation purposes. Through this system, the community mental health agencies provide information relating to characteristics of patients, referral, income, fee, and identification of the presenting problems at time of admission. Termination data include services received, reason for termination, referral if any, and status at time of termination regarding each presenting problem. These data are tabulated and analyzed on both a statewide basis and by agency. The primary value of this system is that it raises questions for further exploration. Specific examples of how this information is used can be seen through the following questions: Is the agency serving a significant number of poor people? Are the fees assessed in accord with the Division of Mental Health's fee schedule? Are there significantly large proportions of patients whose problems are rated other than improved at time of termination? Do large proportions of patients terminate before service has been completed?

The second part of New Hampshire's evaluation system consists of a management by objectives program. This component includes state grant application and reporting procedures. For each program for which an agency seeks state funds, a program plan and budget are presented. These include goals, assessment needs analysis, a statement of quantifiably measurable outcome objectives, and a list of services to be provided. This component includes regular financial and statistical reporting to the Office of Community Mental Health, including information regarding staff time in each program, numbers of patients served, interviews, etc. The service is then broken down into unit costs. Evaluation is conducted by measuring progress toward the mutually agreed upon objectives during the course of the year. Continued state funding for programs depends upon demonstration of satisfactory progress toward the agreed upon objectives. The objectives are still rather primitive, but, then, so are the tools available for measuring progress.

Standards for Community Mental Health Services represent the third part of the evaluation system. Standards for agencies receiving state grants-in-aid have existed for the past ten years. A year ago, with the assistance of the community mental health agencies themselves, these were made more comprehensive. They now refer to such items as minimum qualifications for personnel, physical plant requirements, reporting, intake, fee and personnel policies, requirements for clinical records, etc. The standards, monitored by the central office staff through both agency reports and site visits, represent an effort to ensure a minimum level of competent service to the public.

The fourth portion of the statewide evaluation system is a peer evaluation program that, after having been pilot tested and refined over the past two years, will be formally implemented in Fiscal 1976. Developed with the active assistance of representatives of a number of community mental health agencies in New Hampshire and through consultation with other states—notably Maine and Texas—the plan was to have it begin as a peer consultation, rather than evaluation system. This was because of considerable resistance on the part of some of the community mental health agency executive directors to the idea of having their peers participate in evaluating them. Interestingly, although all the community mental health agency executive directors endorsed the peer consultation concept—to be implemented on a voluntary basis—when it came time for agencies to volunteer to be the consultees, everyone went to the end of the line. Consequently, the Office of Community Mental Health considered the peer site-visit a vital part of a comprehensive evaluation system. To implement this program, staff will be augmented by selected consultants from both within and without New Hampshire's mental health system.

McLean Hospital

McLean Hospital is a 324-bed, private, nonprofit psychiatric hospital located in Belmont, Massachusetts. A teaching hospital of the Harvard Medical School, it was founded as a division of Massachusetts General Hospital.

At McLean, the ultimate objective in evaluation of treatment programming is production and feedback in a manner that will lead to optimal utilization within the system. The appropriate use of evaluative data promotes intervention for more effective and efficient patient care. The Evaluative Service Unit, established in 1972 at McLean Hospital, provides a model for such intervention. As an independent investigatory mechanism it is rather unique in its organizational structure. It is closely linked with selective hospital committees that assume responsibility for review and implementation of evaluative findings. The Unit is established within the hospital as an independent entity to ensure research autonomy. At the same time, a mechanism for ongoing collaboration with the hospital staff enables maximum utilization of research results. This is accomplished through continuous participation of the Evaluative Service Unit team on a hospital committee, known as the Special Studies Subcommittee on Patterns of Patient Care—a satellite of the larger Utilization Review Committee, whose objective includes maintaining high-quality patient care and increasingly effective utilization of hospital services through the use of various review procedures.

Evaluation at McLean is not only an integral part of good clinical practice, but it is also expected to contribute to the process of accountability—both in relation to the organization and to the patient. The major goals of the Unit may be outlined as follows:

1. To carry out relatively brief evaluative studies relating to patient care, as determined by the needs and interests of the hospital.

2. To plan and conduct annually (with the assistance of social work interns as investigators) an extended study relevant to some aspect of patient treatment.
3. To develop an ongoing follow-up program for discharged patients in which both former patients and their families are contacted at predetermined intervals after the patient's hospital discharge (currently at six and eighteen months after discharge).
4. To develop a data bank based on information obtained from all investigations carried out by the Unit for purposes of hospital dissemination.
5. To be available as consultants to hospital staff on matters dealing with evaluative work—including assistance in setting up research designs and/or methodological procedures.
6. To facilitate the feedback process through active contact with clinical units for face-to-face review and interpretation of findings.
7. To prepare reports of all completed studies for professional staff, for publication when feasible, and for wider distribution to the relevant professional community.

A variety of studies and activities are underway by the Evaluative Service Unit. Three of these are described here.[a]

The Follow-up Program

The follow-up program for discharged patients, (excluding those in geriatric, in alcoholism, or in children's units) began, in December 1972, with posthospital intervals for follow-up defined as six months and eighteen months. Both the former patient and a significant relative were included as participants. The first full year of follow-up investigation for the six-month posthospital interval was reported in June 1974. The second was reported in October 1975. Both years of follow-up monitoring met with a response rate of over 80 percent for the patient/family units that were contacted. The more recent investigation provided data on twice as many patient/family units (430 compared to 225), because of the increasing numbers of admissions to the hospital. The methodological approach is primarily by mailed questionnaire, with the supplementation of telephone interviews for nonrespondents to the mailing. Data analysis has been completed for the eighteen-month posthospital interval, for comparison with the six-month data already reported.

Some objectives of the follow-up program include (1) obtaining the former patient's and relative's view of both the posthospital level of functioning and the helpfulness of various aspects of the hospital experience, (2) comparing popula-

[a]The Evaluative Service Unit at McLean has an extensive series of reports, summarizing the results of their studies. Space limitations do not permit a full listing of the full range of studies. Further details may be obtained from the Unit's Director.

tions and outcomes annually, (3) reviewing follow-up data by separate residential halls for dissemination to them, (4) determining emerging patterns or trends that would help to identify high risk populations and necessary modifications of existing service programs. In addition, the type of overview provided by this examination of posthospital careers is expected to highlight areas for further investigation.

Collection of Admission Unit Statistics

Because of the changing size and nature of the hospital population in recent years, the Evaluative Service Unit began to compile statistics on patients admitted to the Admissions Unit that was opened in December 1972. Monthly summaries of statistical data are made available to hospital staff, and two annual reports have been distributed (January 1974 and February 1975). The information collected describes the demographic and clinical characteristics of the patients admitted, as well as their disposition at the time of leaving.

Collection of Discharge Data

The development of a routine data collection system at the time of disposition has been implemented since September 1974 with the cooperation of the After-Care Unit at the hospital. At discharge, the patient is requested to complete a questionnaire to provide baseline information for the postdischarge follow-up questionnaire sent out several months later. These data are currently being collected and will be ready for analysis and comparison, following the completion of posthospital data collection.

Butler Hospital

Butler, a private, nonprofit psychiatric hospital in Rhode Island, has established a Division of Research and Evaluation, the core of which is financed by the operating revenue of that hospital. The Division of Research and Evaluation encompasses the Medical Records Department, Utilization Review and Medical Care Evaluation, and Clinical Research, all of which enhance interaction between research and evaluative and the other divisions of the hospital, including inpatient, outpatient, education and training, and administration and development. Much of the Research and Evaluation staff is also involved in clinical work, thus strengthening the postulate that research and evaluation questions are relevant to important variables in the clinical process.

In addition to development of a management information system for Butler,

Research and Evaluation staff are conducting a variety of studies, two of which are briefly described here and have relevance to the management information system.

Day Hospital as an Alternative or After-care Setting

The first of these two studies is a study of day hospital as an alternative or after-care treatment modality. In order to have a day hospital, Blue Cross must agree to support day-hospital hospitalization as part of its benefit program. After negotiation, Blue Cross agreed to substitute day-hospital days for inpatient days up to the total of the forty-five-day hospitalization allowed by their policy in a calendar year. The study was placed on an experimental basis, with the condition that by the end of the year the effects of the day hospital would be evaluated.

The study design used the population of hospital patients during the first year and divided them into two groups: one group consisted of forty-six patients who went to the day hospital only and did not use the inpatient facilities. The second group included sixty-three patients who had been hospitalized in the inpatient setting first, where day-hospital treatment was used as in after-care setting.

In each of these groups, patients were matched with inpatient controls on the variables of age, sex, diagnosis, major problems, and severity of illness impairment. Thus, each day-hospital-only person was matched with an inpatient-only person who received treatment within the same one-year period. In similar fashion, patients who had experienced day-hospital treatment following inpatient treatment were matched on these variables with patients who had received inpatient treatment to be followed by discharge directly to the community.

Clinical outcome at discharge was measured in three ways: (1) by the clinician's assessment at discharge, (2) by an overall severity-of-impairment rating made by researchers from the discharge summary, and (3) by researchers' ratings of severity of impairment in regard to each specific problem, and a summary of these to yield a total-impairment rating. The comparative results of this study were specific to whether the day hospital was used as an alternative or after-care setting. When the day hospital is used as an after-care setting it is neither more nor less cost-effective than inpatient hospitalization that is not followed by day hospital treatment. The total charges were not different. While inpatient days averaged forty days, inhospital days followed by day-hospital days averaged twenty inpatient days, followed by seventeen day-hospital days. The length of attachment is longer for the inpatient followed by day-hospital treatment (fifty-six days); the inpatient-only length of attachment was forty days. In terms of clinical outcome there were no differences between the two groups. In both modalities over 90 percent were improved at discharge.

When the day hospital was used as an alternative to inpatient treatment, it was found to be clinically as effective, but only half as expensive. Again, in both groups, more than 90 percent were rated as improved at discharge. In terms of treatment costs, day-hospital-only patients were charged an average of $1407. Their inpatient controls were charged $3309, on the average ($p < .001$). In terms of length of stay, day hospital patients used twenty-four day-hospital days, whereas the inpatient matched controls used 36 inpatient days ($p < .001$). However, the length of attachment to the day hospital was longer (sixty days) than the length of attachment of the inpatients (thirty-six days) ($p < .001$).

In summary, when the day hospital was used as an after-care setting following inpatient treatment, it was neither more nor less cost-effective than inpatient treatment only. As an alternative to inpatient treatment, it was just as effective as inpatient treatment and only half as expensive.

Problem Lists as Predictors of Treatment and Outcome

A second study relates more directly to the management information system being developed at Butler—entitled "Problem Lists as Predictors of Treatment and Outcome." The long-term goal of the research is to determine the extent to which the combined use of problem-oriented medical records and systematic posttreatment assessments can provide a mechanism whereby the cost-effectiveness of psychiatric treatments can be routinely assessed and applied to several needs of a mental health treatment system: utilization review, program planning, and clinical research.

Specific aims of the study may be summarized as follows:

1. To develop a classificational system for coding patient problems identified and defined by clinical personnel using the problem-oriented record.

2. To examine the interrelationships among patient problems, in order to identify possible problem clusters.

3. To examine the relationship between identified patient problems and problem clusters, and psychiatric diagnoses.

4. To determine whether problem lists can supplement or supplant psychiatric diagnoses in utilization review studies as predictors of measures of treatment such as treatment costs, types and lengths of stay. Thus utilization studies of patterns of psychiatric care can be established.

5. To conduct systematic assessments of posttreatment outcome so that it will be possible to initiate studies of the interrelationship of pretreatment assessment, and treatment and posttreatment assessments immediately following the completion of the present project.

A satisfactory achievement of the first aim is a prerequisite to the remainder of the study. Without an adequate representation of problem list data, a test of its predictive validity would perform a disservice to the development of problem orientations. The classification scheme should be oriented to problem statements that occur with some frequency, to problems for which treatment interventions are likely, to acceptance by clinical staff of problem classification as valid representations of the problems they have defined, to problem classification in ideal form, and code development guided by both empirical and rational considerations.

Each problem definition is, in principle, idiosyncratic to the patient described. Thus, the task of the problem code to be developed is to capture the significant similarities in problem descriptions so that problem characterizations can be aggregated for quantitative analyses. (Only with recurring events can relationships between these events be established.)

The adequacy of the code is about to be retested empirically. Once its "conceptual/phenomenal fit" is found satisfactory, three years of problem-oriented records will be coded, which will yield a study population of about 3,000 patients. As soon as research money is available, follow-up assessments of this population will be initiated to begin to answer the question of whether, and when, problem lists can be used to supplant diagnoses as predictors of treatment and outcome for psychiatric patients.

List of Contributors

Charles Acker, Ph.D., Project Director, Department of Mental Health and Corrections, Bureau of Mental Health, Augusta, Maine.

David Askew, Ph.D., Director of Mental Health Services, Aroostook Mental Health Center, Fort Fairfield, Maine.

Edgar R. Casper, L.L.M., Krank, Gross, Notturno, and Casper, Harrisburg, Pennsylvania. Former Deputy Attorney General, Commonwealth of Pennsylvania.

Elaine Cumming, Ph.D., Professor of Sociology, University of Victoria, Victoria, British Columbia.

John Cumming, M.D., Professor of Psychiatry, University of British Columbia, Vancouver, British Columbia; former Deputy Commissioner of Mental Health, New York State Department of Mental Hygiene.

Jean Endicott, Ph.D., Codirector, Evaluation Section, Biometrics Research at New York State Psychiatric Institute, New York State Department of Mental Hygiene, and Research Associate, Department of Psychiatry, Columbia University, New York.

William Goldman, M.D., Planning Consultant, San Francisco Department of Health. Former Commissioner of Mental Health, Commonwealth of Massachusetts; former chairperson, National Council of Community Mental Health Centers.

Mollie Grob, S.M., A.C.S.W., Director, Evaluative Service Unit, McLean Hospital, Belmont, Massachusetts.

Marcia Guttentag, Ph.D., President of the Division of Personality and Social Psychology, American Psychological Association; Professor, Harvard University, Cambridge, Massachusetts.

Stuart P. Howell, A.C.S.W., Assistant Director of Mental Health for Community Services, State of New Hampshire, Division of Mental Health, Concord, New Hampshire.

Thomas J. Kiresuk, Ph.D., Director, Program Evaluation Resource Center, Minneapolis, Minnesota.

Richard Longabaugh, Ed.D., Director of Evaluation and Research, Butler Hospital, Providence, Rhode Island and Associate Professor of Medical Sciences, Brown University, Providence, Rhode Island.

Lee B. Macht, M.D., Director of Clinical Services, Cambridge-Somerville Mental Health and Retardation; Associate Director, Department of Psychiatry, Cambridge Hospital and Associate Professor of Psychiatry, Harvard Medical School at the Cambridge Hospital; former interim Commissioner of Mental Health, Commonwealth of Massachusetts.

Robert Spitzer, M.D., Director, Evaluation Section, Biometrics Research, New York State Department of Mental Hygiene at the New York Psychiatric Institute and Associate Professor of Clinical Psychiatry, Columbia University.

Herbert C. Schulberg, Ph.D., Associate Executive Vice President, United Community Planning Corporation, Boston, Massachusetts and Associate Clinical Professor of Psychology, Department of Psychiatry, Harvard Medical School, Boston, Massachusetts.

Gary L. Tischler, M.D., Professor of Clinical Psychiatry, Yale University School of Medicine, New Haven, Connecticut and Director of the Hill-West Haven Division, Connecticut Mental Health Center, New Haven, Connecticut.

Carol H. Weiss, Ph.D., Senior Research Associate, Bureau of Applied Social Research, Columbia University, New York.

About the Editors

Elizabeth Warren Markson is Director of Research and Evaluation, Massachusetts Department of Mental Health and Adjunct Professor, Department of Sociology, State University of New York at Albany. A sociologist, she has published numerous articles in the areas of mental illness, mental health, and aging. Currently, she is conducting research on the process and impact of deinstitutionalization upon mental hospital staff and patients.

David Franklyn Allen is coordinator of the Quality Care Review Team of the Massachusetts Department of Mental Health and Research Fellow in Psychiatry, Massachusetts General Hospital.

Related Lexington Books

Bauman, Gerald, and Grunes, Ruth., *Psychiatric Rehabilitation in the Ghetto: An Educational Approach.* 208 pp., 1974

Foley, Henry, *Community Mental Health Legislation.* 176 pp., 1975

Hollister, Robert M., Kramers, Bernard M., and Bellin, Seymour S., *Neighborhood Health Centers.* 368 pp. 1974

Just, Marion R.; Bell, Carolyn Shaw; Fisher, Walter; and Schensul, Stephen L., *Coping in a Troubled Society: An Environmental Approach to Mental Health.* 128 pp., 1974

Miller, Donald Harlan, *Community Mental Health: A Study of Services and Clients.* 256 pp. 1974

Miller, Mercedese, *Evaluating Community Treatment Programs.* 144 pp., 1975

Smith, Clagett G. and King, James A., *Mental Hospitals: A Study in Organizational Effectiveness.* 208 pp. 1975

Zusman, Jack and Bertsch, Elmer F., *The Future Role of the State Hospital.* 432 pp., 1975

Zusman, Jack and Wurster, Cecil, *Program Evaluation: Alcohol, Drug Abuse, and Mental Health Services.* 320 pp., 1975